Live
Pain-free
without
Drugs or Surgery

Live
Pain-free
without
Drugs or Surgery

How to use
Integrated Positional Therapy
to Eliminate Chronic Pain

Live *Pain-free* without Drugs or Surgery

How to use
Integrated Positional Therapy
to Eliminate Chronic Pain

LEE ALBERT, NMT

Dudley Court Press
Sonoita, AZ

About the Type
This book was set in Adobe Caslon Pro, a typeface originally designed in the 1700s by William Caslon. In the early 1990s Carol Twombly updated the typeface for modern usage.

Cover Image: Dreamstime.com

Published in the United States of America by
Dudley Court Press
PO Box 102
Sonoita, AZ 85637
www.DudleyCourtPress.com

ISBN: 978-0-9831383-1-0

Dedication

To my wife Marcia for her love, support and encouragement

To my publisher Gail for her expertise and dedication

To all my clients who taught me so much

Table of Contents

Appendices

Foreword
By SARK

You and your body are healing geniuses. Let me show you all the ways.

Pain definitely gets my attention and I love finding easy natural solutions for pain relief and whenever possible of course, elimination of pain. I'm writing the foreword for this book because I know through my own physical experience of pain and the absence of pain, that this system – Integrated Positional Therapy – really works. Here's how it worked and continues to work for me:

Some years ago I started a dance practice. After a while, some heel pain developed and then worsened and I started limping because of it. I visited a chiropractor for months, which helped a little but the pain continued. Acupuncture didn't significantly help either.

I started a new stretching regime and when the pain continued with no relief I visited an orthopedic doctor who treats the dancers in the San Francisco Ballet. She watched me walk and diagnosed plantar fasciitis and recommended orthotics, which I started using. Those didn't help either.

I then bought a portable laser device and also began icing my heels after every walk I took. I'm a daily walker and began walking shorter and shorter distances due to the unresolved pain. It was all very disheartening and I felt hopeless and my health was being compromised from my lack of mobility.

That's when I met Lee Albert, NMT at Kripalu, and experienced Integrated Positional Therapy for the first time. In the session, I warned Lee that if he squeezed my heels, the pain was so acute that I might be tempted to punch him. He smiled gently and said, "I can show you how to resolve that in about 90 seconds."

I felt very skeptical but also drawn to his mild mannered, ego-less approach. As he moved my body into various gentle positions, I really couldn't imagine how this could really be effective at all. Then he showed me how to gently bend my foot backwards and hold the position. I felt tempted to push the position further for "greater benefit" and he said very simply, "This is not like stretching."

He said, "I'm like a carpenter. My job is to show you how to be plumb, level and straight. If you like how you feel, you'll do your homework." Then he squeezed my heel and rotated my foot. I waited for the cascade of pain and there were vague, far away remnants of the memory of a pain.

I looked at him and absolutely marveled. He said, "It will take about 10 days to 2 weeks to reset the muscle memory completely, so that there is no pain." Now I was very eager to see how this same principle might work for the rest of my body!

As Lee worked and showed me various positions, he said, "I'll be giving you handouts so that you'll have the visuals to practice with and do your homework. I'm here to show you how to do this for yourself." I immediately doubted that I could do it without him and said so. He replied, "This is not a system where you need me. All you need is yourself and your body and the willingness to practice." Then he added, "old people are not bent over or crooked because they're old. They're that way because they've been crooked longer."

This statement and the system made practical sense to me, but I wasn't experiencing the dramatic release of pain in other parts of my body like I had with my heels. Until I got up off the table. I had a sensation of what I remember about being 7 years old, and realized that it was complete freedom from pain. Even though I had very minor, non-debilitating pain in the rest of my body, I didn't realize how it might feel to be without it. It felt utterly transformative and releasing and I felt like skipping.

Lee patiently explained that there was homework for me to do, and showed me the handouts and explained the main positions. I left his office clutching the papers and grinning at my good fortune. Then I skipped across the wildflower meadow and felt like a commercial for this system. I wanted to call Oprah and everyone else with a giant audience and say, "Let's show this to EVERYBODY!"

Of course I also wanted to share the system with all of my readers too, but there wasn't a book or DVD yet. I told my friends and family and showed them how to do specific positions. I experienced incredible changes in my neck, shoulders and hips, and reveled in feeling pain free in new ways and continued practicing.

I also showed people I didn't know, like the guy who sold me my new car who limped over to hand me the contract and I knew immediately what it was. When I asked him why he was limping, he said: "Yeah — the doctor says plantar fasciitis and I"m also older and heavier, so it's bound to happen." I showed him the 90 second hold for each foot and gave an abbreviated description of Integrated Positional Therapy. The next day, I returned to pick up my new car and this man was running towards me shouting, "No pain! No pain! No limping!!! My God! It really works!!!" He hugged me and asked if there was a book about it so he could learn more. I assured him that one day there would be.

I loved the simple, practical "do it myself" aspect of this new system and began to do my homework daily. It was immediately very clear, and just as Lee had said, when I did the homework, my body felt better. When I didn't, the aches and pains returned. I mostly did the homework — which is about 5 minutes a day — and felt better.

Each year when I returned to teach at Kripalu, I made an appointment to see Lee and learn even more about the system. I also wished for a teacher in San Francisco where I lived to periodically show me more nuances and sometimes work with me too. I knew that Lee trained people in this system, but so far I hadn't found anybody else who knew it. I also wished for a book or a DVD that I could use at home to expand my practice.

I could see that Lee was so occupied showing people how to do Integrated Positional Therapy, that there wasn't necessarily time or energy for him to create a book or DVD. I decided to share that I was an author and would do anything I could to help him publish his book, including write an endorsement or foreword, which he very enthusiastically responded to, and confirmed my thoughts about

His time and energy for creating a book or DVD.

Then the day came when Lee told me that he was working with a publisher on the book!

I prayed that he'd met somebody good that would help him. And he had. That's how this foreword came to be, and now you can experience this system for yourself and share it with others too.

Our bodies are really miraculous healing devices if we just know the right buttons and knobs and if we know the Integrated Positional Release system. And now you will too. Happy practicing and living without pain!

With love, Susan (aka SARK)

Author, Artist, Succulent Wild Woman
HTTP://WWW.PLANETSARK.COM

"A good heart is better than all the heads in the world."

 EDWARD BULWER-LYTTON

Introduction

It was a beautiful summer day. The sun was shining and felt wonderful on my skin. I had recently completed my studies to be a massage therapist. I was driving along the highways of the placid Quebec countryside and slowly pushed on the brake to come to a stop sign. Suddenly in my rear view mirror I saw a car racing towards me. I knew right away that the car wouldn't stop. Smack! I was rear-ended at 60 mph.

Fortunately I was wearing my seat belt and I didn't hit my head on the windshield. I got out of the car, which was a total wreck. I couldn't believe it. I was fine. Nothing broken or bleeding. It was a miracle.

Pretty soon the police came along. They asked me how I was doing. I said I was a little shaken up but thought I was fine. Due to the severity of the crash the officer insisted I go to the emergency room to have a doctor look me over. At the hospital a doctor checked my vital signs, did a few range of motion tests for my neck and said he thought I would be fine.

And I was fine... for three weeks. Then I started to get migraine headaches. I'd had headaches before but never a migraine. These were excruciating! Sights, smells, sounds would set them off. External smells or sounds of bright lights would set them off. I could barely stand it. So after another trip to the doctor it was decided I should start physical therapy. Little did I know that I was going to have these headaches once a week for the next three years.

I spent those three years going to just about every therapist I could find. I was desperate for relief. I spent tens of thousands of dollars and sought out the best therapies I could find – all with no results. Then one day my whole life changed.

I went to a highly recommended therapist who did things in the therapy that were very gentle. At the time I thought the therapy was not going to help because the therapist just didn't do very much. After the session I thanked her and headed home, disappointed again. I knew this wasn't going to work, just like all the other therapies I had tried hadn't worked. Much to my surprise, however, the migraine headaches never returned. How could this be? One session, no deep work and my headaches were gone? Impossible! I had tried almost every kind of therapy you can think of and nothing had worked. How could this gentle, simple therapy do the trick and relieve the horrendous pain I'd been suffering with for over three years — in one short therapy session?

I set out on a quest to find out what this therapy was and how it worked. I wanted to know and I wanted to share it with everyone on the planet.

This book is a result of my quest. I've been practicing and teaching Integrated Positional Therapy now for 25 years, helping thousands of people to enjoy permanent pain relief without surgery or drugs. I hope this book will help you and your loved ones find relief from painful conditions with gentle therapeutic techniques and simple on-going self-care.

Lee Albert
www.LeeAlbert.com
Lenox, Massachusetts
January, 2012

1

The Key to Unlocking Pain

Pain! Everyone experiences pain at some point. Do you know what causes most of your pain? It is simpler than you think. Remember when your mother told you to sit up or stand up straight? Your mother probably didn't know it but good posture is more than just about looking good. Good posture is essential to a healthy, functioning, pain-free body. Most of your pain is caused by poor posture. You are in pain because you are misaligned or… crooked! Even if you think you have good posture you probably don't. Many misalignments are not obvious to the untrained eye.

This may seem too simple but let's look at some examples. Picture a house in your mind. Imagine that the basement of the house is a little lower on one side. In other words the house is crooked. Over time the crooked house develops all sorts of structural problems, i.e. the roof might leak, windows are hard to open, the chimney is leaning, marbles can roll down the floor, etc. The structure of the building is not carrying the load the way it was designed because it is not level. All these problems are cause by one condition. The house is crooked.

You could also imagine a car with its front end out of alignment. The car will run but the tires will have abnormal strain on them because the car is crooked and those tires will wear out very quickly.

The solution in each case is to bring the building or the car back into proper alignment – give the car or the building "good posture" so that the car or the building carries its load the way it was designed to.

Let's apply this to the human body and your pain.

Do you know what the following conditions have in common: sciatica, plantar fasciitis, carpal tunnel, tennis elbow, low back pain, neck pain and most headaches?

At first, they don't seem to have much in common. They occur in different parts of the body and involve different musculoskeletal structures. However, if you step back and look at the body as a whole, you will notice the common element.

This common element is called **muscle imbalance**. This simply means that some muscles are too short and some muscles are too long. Both muscles will feel tight. The short muscle is contracted and tight while the long muscle is like an overstretched rubber band – too long and very tight.

Since every muscle is attached to a bone, these muscle imbalances pull the bones out of alignment. That's what makes you crooked.

Misalignment of the skeletal structure caused by muscle imbalance can cause compressions of the nerves, discs and other structures in the body. It can also cause the fascia to be twisted. Fascia is a band of fibrous connective tissue enveloping, separating, or binding together muscles, organs, and other soft structures of the body. These twists, compressions and tight muscles ultimately lead to less oxygen in the tissues at those areas. The medical term for this condition is ischemia, which means that there is not an adequate supply of blood getting to the tissues. As a result, the tissue is not getting enough oxygen. **It is the lack of oxygen that is actually causing a lot of the pain.**

In a nutshell, muscle imbalances pull the frame of the body (the bones) into misalignment, which then causes pain in the body. The condition of being out of alignment or crooked results in many neuromuscular pain patterns. It is estimated that 80% of all the pain you will experience in your life is due to mechanical problems. Muscles that are either too long or too short are pulling your bones crooked, causing compression and lack of oxygen to the tissues.

When you go to a doctor, you could be diagnosed with any one of hundreds of conditions. In our Western model of medicine, standard treatment for conditions like sciatica, plantar fasciitis, carpal tunnel, tennis elbow, low back pain, neck pain and most headaches involve treating the symptoms, typically with a pain killer or an anti-inflammatory drug. Seldom does treatment address the cause. The cause is muscle imbalance or misalignment and the correct treatment is to get you "uncrooked."

Integrated Positional Therapy

Integrated Positional Therapy (IPT) is based upon the osteopathic techniques of Strain/Counterstrain and Muscle Energy Technique. Strain/Counterstrain slackens a muscle and makes it shorter while Muscle Energy Technique stretches a muscle and makes it longer.

Don't worry about the technical terms. These techniques are simply used to bring your body back into alignment and out of pain very gently and quickly. Muscle Energy Technique (MET) and Strain/Counterstrain are used to correct the imbalances in the muscles.

MET is a very powerful tool to quickly and easily lengthen tight, constricted muscles and restore range of motion. It is a form of assisted stretching using active isometric contractions.

Strain/Counterstrain can also be applied to these tight, constricted muscles. With this technique, the affected area is passively shortened and held for two minutes, thereby allowing the muscle fibers to effectively reset and return to neutral. The results are often dramatic and long-lasting.

One of the first principles therapists and doctors learn is that the body, including the muscular/

skeletal system, is always trying to achieve homeostasis. This means that it is trying to get back into balance or alignment. The great thing is that we are actually doing this every day. Here's an example. Do you ever lie down on your back and instinctively put your hands under your head? You probably don't think about the movement. You do it because it feels good; your body makes you do it. Why? Because your body is trying to get back into balance. This movement releases and rebalances the shoulders and part of the neck.

Try this experiment for yourself:

Place your left hand on your right shoulder. If you are wearing a shirt you might find a seam in the shirt in this area. With your left hand press somewhere along the seam. This will be tender or sore in many people. Once you have found a tender spot, take your right hand and gently rest it on top of your head. Now press the spot that was sore before. Does it feel better? It usually does. Now hold your right arm in this position on top of your head for two minutes. This period allows the muscle memory to reset. After two minutes, put your right arm back down at your side. Press the tender spot again. It should feel better. The effects of this technique are cumulative, so each time it gets better and better.

Here is another example. Do you ever sit in a chair and cross your legs? Almost everyone does this and yet we don't generally think about it. Our bodies make us cross our legs because the position feels good. The body is trying to achieve homeostasis or balance by gently stretching the outside of the hip and leg. When your body is in balance, it just plain feels good. (Common wisdom is that crossing your legs while sitting in a chair is bad for you, but it is simply the body's way of stretching the muscles on the outside of the leg and hip to bring them back into balance.) When your muscles are in balance, you will no longer cross your legs because it is not needed anymore.

Your body is always trying to heal itself. All you have to do is learn how to listen to it. The body has great wisdom. Whenever your body is telling you one thing and your brain is telling you something else, always listen to the body. The brain can make up some pretty good stories that are not necessarily true.

Positional Therapy is the therapy that cured my migraines. I developed *Integrated* Positional Therapy (IPT) by adding critical components to make the therapy even more effective in relieving chronic pain. IPT is what I now practice and want to share with you in this book. In addition to the basic muscle release techniques of Positional Therapy, Integrated Positional Therapy includes very important exercises to straighten the pelvis and adds Wellness Plans to enhance the immediate and long-term results.

Integrated Positional Therapy (IPT) is designed to eliminate pain at its root cause and not just hide the symptoms. As a self-care technique, this therapy can help you to correct the muscle imbalances in your own body.

With some easy-to-learn practices, you will learn to correct the imbalances by making your short muscles longer and your long muscles shorter. This process will bring your body into alignment and out of pain.

IPT can eliminate the pain associated with many common conditions such as headaches and migraines, back and neck pain, carpal tunnel syndrome, limited range of motion and sports injuries, thoracic outlet syndrome, sciatica, repetitive motion injuries, fibromyalgia, tendonitis, plantar fasciitis and many more. This book covers eleven of the most common conditions. In some cases, a session with a trained Integrated Positional Therapist may be advisable, but most people will find great relief from chronic muscle pain by following the appropriate Wellness Plan described in this book.

Simple, easy-to-do-at-home exercises and other lifestyle habits will maintain the results. On-going maintenance is crucial to keeping your body pain-free. Remember the car analogy? Just as your car needs regular maintenance to stay in great working order, your body requires maintenance to stay pain-free.

The treatment protocols described in this manual are based upon 25 years of clinical experience treating tens of thousands of people with superior results. In the pages that follow, you will learn how to correct your own muscle imbalances. You will learn exactly what is causing your pain. You'll learn how to improve the quality of your life by reducing or eliminating the pain in your body that you are currently enduring. You will also learn some general tips on how to be healthier than you are now. Everything I am going to show you is easy and takes very little time to do. No previous experience is needed. No special equipment is necessary. These practices are designed to fit your busy lifestyle. As a matter of fact, many of the practices can be done in bed, on the couch or at the office.

So let's get started!

2

The Basic Care of Your Body

In order for the body to function at peak health, there are two vital "nutrients" that must be consumed in adequate amounts. These are oxygen and water. Usually these are not given much thought, but they are involved in almost every function of the body. Without these two nutrients, life cannot exist. Pain levels are usually much higher when these two nutrients are not in adequate supply. When there is enough oxygen and water, it is then crucial to get them to the cells. This task is accomplished through circulation. Exercise is, of course, the best way to increase your circulation so your cells can receive all that life-giving, pain-reducing oxygen and water. In this chapter, you will find simple practices to help increase your water and oxygen levels and improve their delivery to the cells of your body.

Oxygen

If you ask people what is the most important ingredient for good health, you will seldom receive the right answer. The most common answers are plenty of water or nutritious food. Both of those are important, but not nearly as important as oxygen. Think about it. People can live thirty days with no food and still will not die. People can live five days with no water and still be alive. However, five minutes with no oxygen causes death. Clearly oxygen is the most important factor in achieving good health and a pain-free body.

Most people do not get enough oxygen. This is mainly due to the fact that we breathe very shallowly. By that, I mean we are using only a small part of our lungs. This is what is referred to as chest breathing. Proper breathing by using all of the lungs starts with the abdominal area filling up with air and then the chest. Most people just fill up the chest, which is about a third of lung capacity. This amount will keep you alive but does not provide enough oxygen for optimal health.

Another reason that we do not get enough oxygen is that there is not as much as there once was in the air we breathe. When scientists measure the percentage of oxygen in the air in a pristine environment such as a country setting with lots of trees and very few cars, the measurement of oxygen tends to be in the mid 20% range. When they measure the oxygen content in an air sample from a big city with few trees and many cars, the oxygen percentage is in the mid teens. Oxygen samples from inside buildings are even worse. They can be as low as 10%.

What is even more eye-opening is that when scientists took ice samples from 3,000 years ago and measured the oxygen content of the air bubbles, they found that it was about 40%. As we continue to cut down trees and pollute the air, we are slowly depriving ourselves of the most vital nutrient on the planet.

Aside from keeping us alive, why is oxygen so important? Low levels of oxygen are associated with all sorts of chronic diseases. Oxygen helps to clean the blood of bacteria and viruses. Oxygen gives you more energy and boosts the immune system. Higher levels of oxygen are usually accompanied by better overall heath.

80% of all the pain people experience in their lives is muscular pain caused by muscle imbalances. The reason that not every tight muscle causes pain has to do with the amount of oxygen the tissues are receiving. When tissues do not get enough oxygen, they hurt a lot more than tissues that are getting enough oxygen. Even if you have a tight muscle, as long as you are getting a lot of oxygen, the oxygen will reduce or eliminate the pain.

The easiest way to get more oxygen is to develop a daily practice of deep, slow breathing. This is easy to do and has many benefits such as reduced pain levels, clearer thinking, more energy, reduced blood pressure and reduced stress levels, to name a few. Do the following exercise at least twice a day for 10-15 minutes and for shorter durations during the day. It may take some practice to break the habit of chest breathing, but it is well worth the effort.

Daily Practice:

Sit up straight or lie on your back.

Place a hand on your abdomen and slowly inhale through your nose.

As you inhale make sure that you feel your abdomen expanding against your hand.

After your abdomen is full continue to inhale so now you feel your chest expanding. This should all be done with no effort or straining.

Slowly exhale through your nose or mouth.

Repeat the process.

Water

Water is critical for all body functions. Experts agree that the body is between 60–70% water. In my opinion, most people are dehydrated — not clinically dehydrated, but enough to cause some serious problems. Proper hydration is the key to all of the body's critical systems. Good health is almost impossible if your cells are not hydrated properly. Signs of dehydration include fatigue, dizziness, constipation, arthritis, headaches, high blood pressure, anxiety and dark-colored urine.

Water is so important that one of the first procedures a doctor will do when you are admitted to the hospital is to give you intravenous saline solution to help you quickly hydrate. Doctors know that good hydration is crucial to good health and reduced muscle pain.

We lose a lot of water just through breathing. If you are out on a cold day, you can see the water vapor with every breath. If you live in a cold climate and live in a heated house, the typical humidity is 15–20%. That is considered desert conditions. Breathing dry air can also lead to dehydration.

Remember that caffeine and alcohol are diuretics and thus take water out of the body. These types of drinks will not hydrate but rather dehydrate and should be consumed in moderation. Drink a little extra water after consuming drinks with caffeine or alcohol.

As the body starts to get low on water, it has to manage this crisis. The body has a system of priority as to how it uses its water. The main priority is the brain. The body does not want the brain to get low on water. If the body is not getting enough water, it has to take it from other places to send to the brain to keep it functioning well.

One of the places the body takes the water from is the joints. As a result, there will not be enough lubrication in the joints, which will cause them to ache and be painful. The body also takes water from the discs between the vertebrae. This can cause the body to get shorter and possibly compress a nerve, which is very painful. The body also takes water from the muscles to send to the brain. This reallocation can cause the muscles to ache more and be less flexible. When the body can no longer get enough water to send to the brain, symptoms such as memory loss, brain fog and headaches can occur.

How much water and fluids should a person consume every day? The key is not how much you drink but how much your cells absorb. This amount can depend on many factors. In general:

- Water is better absorbed when it is sipped slowly and not guzzled.
- It is also better absorbed when it is warm or hot.
- If you are not on a salt-restricted diet, you will also absorb more water if you add a pinch of sea salt to the water. The minerals in the salt let the cells take in more water.
- Coconut water is also excellent for rehydrating the body.

Daily Practice:

Have a glass of room temperature water upon awakening to replace the fluids lost during sleep.

Sip water or herbal tea all day long.

Carry a water bottle with you when you are not home so you have a water supply.

Be consistent. It takes up to 6 weeks to rehydrate.

Try to consume half of your body weight in ounces of water. For example, if you weigh 150 pounds try consuming 75 ounces of fluid a day. Build up to these levels slowly so as not to overtax your bodily systems.

If you are taking a diuretic, check with your doctor first before rehydrating.

Exercise

It is well known that people who exercise are usually healthier and have more energy. One of the reasons for their superior health is that they are getting more water and oxygen to their cells through increased blood flow. Blood delivers oxygen and water to the cells, which increases energy and decreases pain.

Exercise raises your heart rate. The heart is the pump that circulates your blood. The better the circulation, the more energy you have and the less pain you experience. Even if you have sore muscles, often just a twenty-minute walk will raise the heart rate enough to reduce the pain.

Exercise also contributes to better mental focus and a reduced chance of suffering from depression. Exercise stimulates brain chemicals that can make you happier and more relaxed. Exercise also helps to prevent or reverse osteoporosis. It will also improve your digestion, increase your metabolism and help you to sleep better. Exercise helps to manage your cholesterol and helps to prevent Type 2 Diabetes. With all these benefits, it is certainly worthwhile to include some exercise in your life daily.

Many people lead a sedentary life. They wake up in the morning, drive to work, sit at work all day, drive home, watch TV and then go to bed. That is a recipe for painful, weak muscles, depression and/or brain fog, unhealthy weight levels and sleepless nights. The old adage "use it or lose it" is true. Before exercising, of course check with your doctor and see if you are fit to do so. There is no need for fancy equipment or expensive gyms, although those are fine. Simple walking will do. The human body was designed to walk many miles a day back when we were hunter-gatherers. Start with just 10 minutes of walking a day if that is where your fitness level feels comfortable. The main thought to keep in mind is not to do too much too soon. Moderation is the key. Daily exercise that raises your heart rate even just a little will bring tremendous benefits to your physical and mental state of being.

Daily Practice:

Walk or do some gentle exercise that raises the heart rate for 20–30 minutes a day.

Rebounding on a mini trampoline is also an excellent form of exercise that is easy on the joints.

Increase the time slowly as your fitness level improves.

3

What's Your Pain Problem?
Symptoms and Conditions Check-in

Check the following chart to find the condition that most closely describes your symptoms. It does not need to be a perfect match.

Test for the condition until you confirm which condition is creating your symptoms. If none of the tests confirm a particular condition, choose the Wellness Plan for the condition that is most closely associated with your symptoms. If you have several conditions, choose the Wellness Plan for the dominant or primary condition to start.

IF THESE ARE YOUR SYMPTOMS	YOU MAY SUFFER FROM	DO THIS TEST TO CONFIRM
Sensation of pain, tightness or pressure around the forehead or back of the head and neck. The pain is sometimes described as throbbing or aching and can affect the front, top or side of the head.	Tension-Type Headaches	No test is necessary. If you have persistent headaches, see your health care provider as this could be a sign of a more serious problem.
Sensation of pain in the neck that could be described as an ache, stiffness, burning or stabbing. This condition can be acute or chronic. It is often better in certain positions such as lying down or standing.	Neck Pain	Bend your head in different directions. If there is pain, stiffness or aching, this could be neck pain or tight, sore muscles that could be a precursor to the condition.

IF THESE ARE YOUR SYMPTOMS	YOU MAY SUFFER FROM	DO THIS TEST TO CONFIRM
Sensation of pain with sounds such as clicking, grating, and/or popping. Can also cause headaches and earaches and make it difficult to open your mouth wide.	TMJ (Temporomandibular Joint Disorder)	With the mouth open, press on the joint near the ear. If this is painful, this could be TMJ or tight, sore muscles that could be a precursor to the condition. If you cannot open your mouth very wide, or it is painful to do so, this could also be TMJ.
Sensation of pain, numbness, tingling, weakness or coldness in the arm and/or hand.	Thoracic Outlet Syndrome (TOS)	Raise both hands over your head with fingers pointing toward the ceiling and palms facing straight ahead. Rapidly open and close hands. Do this for 1 minute. If there is numbness, tingling or coldness within the minute, this could be TOS or tight, sore muscles that could be a precursor to the condition.

IF THESE ARE YOUR SYMPTOMS	YOU MAY SUFFER FROM	DO THIS TEST TO CONFIRM
Sensation of pain or discomfort at the site of the elbow, sometimes radiating to other parts of the arm.	Tennis or Golfer's Elbow (Medial or Lateral Epicondylitis)	Hold your right arm out in front of you with elbow straight and palm facing down. With the left hand, bend the right wrist so that the fingers on the right hand are pointing toward ceiling. Then bend the right hand at the wrist down toward the floor so the fingers are pointing down. If this causes pain on the outside of the elbow, it could be tennis elbow. If this causes pain on the inside of the elbow, this could be golfer's elbow or tight, sore muscles that could be a precursor to the condition. Test the other side.

IF THESE ARE YOUR SYMPTOMS	YOU MAY SUFFER FROM	DO THIS TEST TO CONFIRM
Sensation of pain, numbness, tingling, burning or weakness in the hand and fingers.	Carpal Tunnel Syndrome (CTS)	Test for CTS on the right hand. From a normal standing position with your arms at your side, bend your right elbow to 90° with your palm facing down. Use your left hand to gently push your left hand toward the floor, creating a bend in the wrist. If pain, numbness, tingling, burning or weakness develop within a minute, this could be CTS or tight, sore muscles that could be a precursor to the condition. Test on the other side.
Sensation of pain in the lower back that could be described as an ache, stiffness, burning or stabbing. This condition can be acute or chronic. It is often better in certain positions such as lying down or standing.	Low Back Pain	Bend your body in different directions. If there is pain, stiffness or aching, this could be low back pain or tight, sore muscles that could be a precursor to the condition.

IF THESE ARE YOUR SYMPTOMS	YOU MAY SUFFER FROM	DO THIS TEST TO CONFIRM
Sensation of pain, numbness, tingling or weakness that you feel in your back or buttocks and down your leg and sometimes may move into your foot.	Sciatica or Piriformis Syndrome	Sit upright on the edge of a chair. Place one ankle on the opposite thigh. Keeping the back straight, bend forward at the waist while bringing your chest toward your knee. If this movement increases the numbness or tingling, this could be Piriformis Syndrome. If the pain is just in the buttocks, this could be a tight piriformis. If you cannot get into this position, this is due to tight muscles that may lead to this condition. Repeat on the other side. **If at any time the pain is too severe to attempt this test, call your doctor for evaluation.**
Sensation on the inside of the knee that is painful to the touch, often accompanied by swelling.	Medial Knee Pain (Medial Meniscus strain or tear)	Sit cross-legged, yoga-style. If this causes pain on the inside of the knee, this could be a Medial Meniscus strain or tear or tight, sore muscles that could be a precursor to the condition. If you cannot get into this position, this is due to tight muscles that may lead to this condition. Repeat on the other side. **For severe, acute pain of the knee, first seek evaluation by your physician.**

IF THESE ARE YOUR SYMPTOMS	YOU MAY SUFFER FROM	DO THIS TEST TO CONFIRM
Sensation of pain in the heel or the bottom of the foot.	Plantar Fasciitis	If the pain in the heel or bottom of the foot is worse in the morning and improves throughout the day or the pain is worse when you are walking without shoes, it could be plantar fasciitis or tight, sore muscles that could be a precursor to the condition.
Sensation of chronic, widespread pain with tenderness to light touch. This often occurs with fatigue. There can be tingling of the skin that feel like needles. There may also be nerve pain and brain fog.	Fibromyalgia	Pain must be on both the left and right sides of the body and both above and below the waist. This may also just be tight, sore muscles or dehydration.

4

Overview of
Integrated Positional Therapy Wellness Plans

In the following chapters, you will find definitions of each condition to aid you in understanding the mechanics of the condition that is causing your pain. Remember that all of these conditions are caused by certain muscles being too long and tight and some being too short and tight. These tight muscles pull the bones out of alignment, which can cause muscle pain, disc problems, nerve compressions and tendonitis.

You will also find a list of common causes for each of these conditions. In order for the body to feel better, it is important not only to reduce or eliminate the pain but also to eliminate the cause. This process often involves doing your daily activities in a slightly different way that stops the pain from returning. The old saying "If you do what you always did, you get what you always got" applies here.

In my 25 years of helping people, I have identified three activities that almost everybody does and which cause 50–60% of all the pain I treat. These activities are: sitting in a chair, sitting in a car and sitting at a computer. It is not the computer or the chair or the car causing the pain but the way you are using those instruments. If you just do these three things a little differently, half of your pain can be eliminated. In the following pages, I will show you how easy it is to obtain good results and how beneficial they can be.

Most people have the same or similar muscular imbalances in their bodies. This coincidence is explained by the fact that we do similar activities all day long. For example, most of us drive a car, sit at a computer or slump in our chairs for a good part of the day. These positions will bring about similar muscular aches and pains. Almost everyone has tight neck muscles, whether they hurt or not. Neck tightness is caused by slumping over the computer or steering wheel or just walking with your head forward of the body. These positions all cause the neck to be tight.

Almost everyone also has a pelvis that is out of balance, i.e. crooked. It is crucial that the pelvis be brought back into balance. There are three ways the pelvis is usually out of balance.

1) One hip is higher than the other. This then looks like one leg is shorter. Although the leg is not truly shorter, it is functionally shorter when walking, which puts undue strain on the body structure.

2) The pelvis is rotated. If you lie on your back on the floor and your feet turn way out, your hip is rotated. This puts a lot of strain on the low back and the knees.

3) The pelvis is tilted either forward or backward. This imbalance will give you an exaggerated curve in your low back and also puts undo strain on the entire body structure.

Most people will have at least one of these imbalances and many have all three. I provide three stretches which usually bring the pelvis back into balance.

The treatment protocols listed for each condition evolved over 25 years to ensure safe, effective, easy application and were designed to fit your busy schedule. They only take minutes a day and will give you the tools to effectively deal with your muscular pains. Some of these protocols are about prevention and some are proactive in ridding yourself of the pain. It is important that they are done consistently and gently. None of these stretches should hurt.

Caution: Never stretch into a painful position. You will achieve better results by being gentle.

Our goal is not to stretch as far as possible but to slightly increase range of motion. When the exercises are done every day, the results can be dramatic and permanent.

You will notice that many of the protocols are similar. Most of them include the three hip stretches to balance the pelvis. Whether it is a pain in the foot or the head, the root cause is often a crooked pelvis.

I want to take some time now to further discuss slackening a muscle. Most of us are familiar with stretching a muscle, but we don't often think about slackening a muscle. A good analogy is to think of a string. If I take the two ends of a string and pull them farther apart, this is called stretching. Slackening a muscle is taking the two ends of the string and bringing them closer together. This gives the muscle slack. If there is slack, there is no tension. If there is no tension, there is no pain. That position of slack must be held for two minutes in order for the muscle memory to take effect and keep the muscle loose. The result often feels like a miracle, as the pain just seems to disappear.

Remember the exercise on page 3? That was a demonstration of putting a muscle in slack. Try it again now:

Take your left hand and gently put it on your right shoulder. Find a seam on your shirt that runs toward your neck. Somewhere along that seam, press into the tissue with a finger on your left hand. You will probably feel that it is sore, bumpy or tight. This indicates a muscle imbalance in the region. Now keep your left hand where it is but stop pressing the tissue. Take your right arm and gently rest your forearm on top of your head. Completely relax it in that position. With your left hand, press the tissue again. It should feel softer and less painful. If it still hurts, move the arm into slightly different positions until the tissue feels better. You just put that muscle into slack.

Holding it in that position for two minutes lets the muscle "reset" itself.

These protocols are designed to treat the whole body and not just the site of the pain. By treating the whole body and removing the root, Integrated Positional Therapy obtains longer-lasting results.

How Soon Can I Expect Results?

In most cases of pain caused by muscle imbalances, relief is immediate. Rebalancing the muscles usually gives a muscle 80–100% relief almost immediately and the effects are cumulative. The more you do it, the better the results.

If the muscle imbalances have been there a long time, sometimes inflammation is present. The Wellness Plan will rebalance the muscles, but it could take 1–2 weeks for the inflammation to clear up.

If dehydration is a factor in your muscle pain, it could take 6–8 weeks for the pain to get better, as that is how long it takes to rehydrate the body.

Finally, although the protocols in this manual are very effective, sometimes medical attention is required. *If the protocols are not working or you are getting worse, please go see your health care provider.*

5

Tension Type Headache and Migraine

Headache is one of the most common reasons people seek medical help. It is estimated that in the United States alone we spend between $50–70 billion on headaches every year. That figure includes medical visits, alternative therapies and over-the-counter pain medication.

Recent research shows that most headaches are probably a combination of tension and migraine. Whether the headache is caused by the muscle tension or the muscle tension results from the headache, treating that muscle tension can provide significant relief from the pain.

Tension type headaches are often due to muscle imbalances in the neck and shoulder muscles. This means the tight muscles are either too long or too short and are pulling or compressing other structures in this area, that can lead to the pain. Even though the pain is experienced in the head, the cause is often in the neck or shoulder area.

Many migraine headaches are also aggravated by muscle imbalances, but some are not. Other factors for migraine are diet, brain chemical imbalances and hormonal imbalances. This chapter addresses migraines and headaches caused by muscle imbalances. *If the protocols listed in this book are not working, check with your health care provider, as you might have a migraine not caused by muscle imbalances or dehydration.*

You can improve or eliminate your headaches with a little awareness and some self-care. It is vital to first identify and correct the common everyday activities that are the source of muscle strain in the neck and shoulders that can lead to a headache. There are many things you do every day that may lead to pain and spasm in the muscles of the head, neck, or shoulders.

We all have demands that keep us working through our pain. So we continually re-strain the area through our daily activities until we learn how to do those activities without causing muscle strain. The protocols listed in this book will help you perform your daily activities with little or no pain or show you how to relieve the pain that occurs because of these activities. Our plan is to reduce or eliminate as many causes of muscle strain as we can and apply stretches or slackenings to correct the muscle imbalances.

One of the most common causes of these muscle imbalances is simply poor posture and/or improper ergonomics. Slumping at your desk or in your car pushes your head forward of your body, putting a lot of strain on your neck and shoulders, which now have to hold up your head without the support of the spinal column. The average head weighs between 8–12 pounds. That is very heavy. If you tried to hold that much weight with your arms, you probably would not last more than five minutes. Yet we ask our neck and shoulder muscles to hold that weight all day long. These muscles are not designed to hold up your head. They are meant to move your head in different directions, not hold it in the same position for long periods of time. By correcting your computer and driving positions, you will bring your head over your shoulders, giving yourself good posture. Your bones (the spinal column) will be holding up your head, which will help take the strain off the muscles.

Another major factor in the cause of headaches is the lack of water. In my opinion, many people do not drink enough water to adequately hydrate their cells. Muscles that do not get enough water ache more than muscles that are well hydrated. Remember that caffeine and alcohol are diuretics, which means they take water out of the body. It is fine to have these things in moderation, but remember to drink even more water afterward. People will overlook the basics like drinking water and this is often the cause of many aches and pains. If you feel a headache coming on, immediately drink two large glasses of water. Prompt fluid intake will often stop the headache. In general, drink half your body weight in ounces every day. This will help reduce the frequency of your headaches and lead to better overall health. It can take up to six weeks to rehydrate, so please be patient.

It is also very important to stretch the neck muscles every day. Many people have a head-forward posture, which will put quite a strain on the neck muscles. A tight neck can lead to a headache. Many people walk into my office rubbing their neck and saying that they hold all their stress in their neck. While this is true, it is not the kind of stress most people think. It is not so much "I got a ticket," "the boss yelled at me," or "the car broke down." This kind of emotional stress can of course add to the tension and pain in the neck and head. The real source, however, is mostly a mechanical stress of having the head and/or arms forward of the body when either sitting or standing. Bad posture is responsible for a great amount of the stress in the neck that can lead to a headache.

By adopting the Wellness Plan in this chapter, you can eliminate or significantly reduce the number and severity of your headaches. If after practicing the Wellness Plan you still have no improvement, see your health care provider for further assessment.

Symptoms:

A tension headache is felt as pain, tightness or pressure around the head. The pain is sometimes described as throbbing or aching and can affect the front, top, back or side of the head. The pain can be felt in the neck, upper back, eyes, jaw or other muscle groups in the body. It may also radiate from other areas like the shoulders or upper back.

Common Causes:

There are many lifestyle habits that can contribute to a headache. The following are some of the most common I have come across in my practice.

- Poor posture, especially head forward of the body or arms held extended for long periods of time. These postures are typical of driving and computer positions. They put a lot of strain on the neck and shoulder muscles that can lead to a headache.

- Emotional or mental stress, anxiety, TMJ and/or teeth grinding at night. This kind of stress makes your tight muscles even tighter. Try the breathing exercise described in Chapter 2.

- Fatigue and/or lack of sleep. Fatigue upsets the chemical balance in the body and can lead to a headache. Try to get 7-8 hours of uninterrupted sleep.

- Dehydration. Lack of water can make your joints and/or muscles ache a lot more. (See Chapter 2 for instructions for proper hydration.)

- Eyestrain. Eyestrain can cause a headache due to muscle imbalances around the eye. If you wear glasses, make sure your prescription is up to date; if you do not wear glasses, see your eye doctor, as you might need them. Periodically give your eyes a rest. While at the computer, take a break and stare out the window for a few minutes. This shift in attention gives the eye a different focal point and helps to relieve eye strain.

- Caffeine withdrawal. When giving up caffeine, always do so slowly. Slowly coming off caffeine and keeping well hydrated can mitigate the effects of withdrawal.

- Hunger. Low blood sugar can also lead to a headache. Eat a balanced diet at regular intervals to keep the blood sugar even. Do not skip meals. Protein helps to keep blood sugar levels more even.

- Reading in bed with head propped up. This is a common practice that leads to a lot of headaches. This position really strains the neck and shoulder muscles.

With a little awareness and by following the Wellness Plan in this book, you can easily make the changes in your life that will help stop your headaches from returning.

Conventional Medical Approach

Standard medical treatments for headaches often include pain-killers, muscle relaxants and anti-depressants. Remember that these drugs do not cure headaches; rather, they hide the symptoms for a while. They are not addressing two of the biggest factors of headaches – dehydration and muscle imbalances.

IPT WELLNESS PLAN FOR TENSION-TYPE HEADACHE & MIGRAINE

MUSCLE RE-BALANCING: This section explains the exercises you need to do to correct the muscle imbalances that are causing your pain. By doing these exercises now, and continuing to do them as instructed, you will make your short muscles longer and your long muscles shorter and bring them back into balance.

Three Stretches to Balance the Pelvis (Appendix B)

These stretches will help to bring the body structure back into balance, thus eliminating a major cause of aches and pains. These exercises are designed to stretch the muscles or muscle groups that are typically too short in most people and are pulling the pelvis out of alignment. When the pelvis is crooked, this affects all the areas of the body. A pelvis that is out of alignment is often a major cause of neck strain and thus headaches, as many headaches are caused by tight neck muscles. Do these stretches twice a day.

Three Neck Stretches (Appendix C)

These stretches will loosen the muscles in the neck and shoulders and allow more blood and oxygen to flow to the head and neck. It takes about 90 seconds to do these stretches and doing them is a great habit to cultivate, as you will feel less pain and stiffness in the neck and you will be more alert. Consistent practice will reduce or eliminate the cause of many headaches. Gently stretch the neck muscles three times a day.

Slacken the Jaw (Appendix D)

Slackening the jaw will help to loosen the masseter muscle in the jaw, which is usually very tight and short in most people. This tight muscle can refer pain to the head and/or pull the jaw out of alignment which can then lead to a headache. Do this five times a day until the symptoms subside.

Slacken the Shoulders (Levator scapula & upper trapezius) (Appendix E)

Slackening the shoulders will relieve tension in the shoulders, especially the upper trap and levator scapula muscle. These areas are tight and sore in most people. Do this exercise any time you feel any tension in your shoulders or neck and at least five times a day. Do not do this exercise if it hurts to put your arm on top of your head.

Shoulder Shrugs (Appendix E)

Shoulder shrugs will help relax your shoulder and neck muscles and bring more blood and oxygen to the area, which will reduce tension and pain. This will also help you feel more alert. Repeat several times throughout the day.

Strengthen Rhomboids (Appendix E)

Strengthening the rhomboids will help to shorten and strengthen the muscles between the shoulder blades, thus training the muscles to bring the head over the shoulders, improving the posture and reducing the strain on the neck. Do this ten times, three times a day.

Stretch the Chest (Pectoralis Major & Minor) (Appendix F)

In most people the chest muscles are too short and the rhomboids between the shoulder blades are too long, which give a person a head-forward, bent-over look with rounded shoulders. Stretching the chest muscles will release tension between the shoulder blades and open up the chest, which will make a person stand up straighter. When a person stands straight, the bones in the cervical spine hold up the head and the neck muscles can relax. Hold for at least two minutes. Do this exercise twice a day.

Slacken the Chest (Appendix F)

Slackening the chest muscles will relax the muscles in the chest, especially the pectoralis minor muscle. Relaxing these muscles helps people with shoulders rounded forward to bring them back into better alignment and will help to bring the head over the shoulder, thus reducing strain on the neck. Totally relax and hold that position for two minutes. Do this twice a day.

SUPPORTIVE LIFESTYLE: This part of your Wellness Plan is designed to address the root of the problem and to relieve habitual muscle imbalances to avoid aggravating the condition as you go about your daily life.

Check Sitting, Driving And Computer Positions (Appendix A)

Correcting your posture while sitting, driving and working at a computer will ensure the pelvis stays in balance and that you are not causing more stress on the neck, shoulders and lower and upper back. These common activities are responsible for a great amount of the pain in your life.

Doing these activities the wrong way will make your body crooked and lead to muscle imbalances that could lead to a headache and possible lumbar or cervical disc problems. By slightly changing the way you perform these activities, you will keep the body in alignment and help ensure that once the pain is relieved it does not come back. Remember if you do what you always did, you get what you always got.

Walk or Stand Holding Your Wrist Behind Your Back

This stance will ensure that you have good posture when you are standing or walking. It will bring the head over the shoulders, open the chest and correct any pelvic tilt. This position should be used when you are walking slowly or standing in one place. When walking briskly, swing your arms naturally, which will help to move and clean out your lymphatic system, which is the body's sewer system.

Keep Elbows Close To Body When Performing Daily Activities

Holding the arms away from the body for long periods can lead to tight sore muscles in many areas of your body and cause a headache. In addition to your driving and computer positions, other common activities that cause muscle strain are using the phone and household activities like chopping vegetables or vacuuming. Performing your daily activities with your elbows close by your side will eliminate or prevent a lot of your pain.

Stay Well Hydrated

One of the most common causes of headache is dehydration. Even slight dehydration can cause a headache. Many people are dehydrated. If the headache is just starting, immediately drink two large glasses of water. This will often help. If you already have a headache, start hydrating as soon as possible. See page 8 for instructions on how to drink water and how much. It can take up to six weeks to rehydrate.

Keep The Neck As Warm As Possible

Wear a collar, turtleneck shirt or scarf around your neck, even inside the house. Keeping the neck as warm as possible will help keep the neck loose and reduce the pain. A cold breeze on the neck is a factor in many headaches and stiff necks.

Regular Exercise

Light regular exercise such as walking every day for at least 20 minutes can help with your headache by increasing your circulation. Exercise also releases certain neurotransmitters (chemicals) in the brain that can help eliminate pain.

Heat shoulders and neck for 20 minutes

Use a heating pad on the neck and shoulders every day for about 20 minutes. Applying warmth will help to relax the muscles in the area and bring more blood and oxygen to the tissues. Continue until the symptoms subside.

Success Story

A 37-year-old woman came to me for help with her headaches. She had suffered from these headaches for about five years. They would occur about once a week. On a pain scale of 1-10, her headaches were a 7 or 8. She was following her doctor's advice and treating them with over-the-counter pain medications. She did not have a headache the day I saw her. They occurred mostly on the right side of her head in the temple, forehead and behind the eye. Headaches in this area almost always originate in the upper trap muscles on the top of the shoulder. I needed to find out what she was doing to make this muscle so tight that it produced a headache.

The upper trap muscle gets tight with any head-forward posture, typically driving or sitting at a computer the wrong way. Sure enough, she had a desk job. I asked her to describe her workstation set-up. She showed me how she sat at her computer. Her head was far forward while looking at her screen, which was too low, and her arm was extended far away from her body to hold the mouse. The entire posture was putting tremendous strain on the upper trap muscle. When I touched the muscle, it was very sore to the touch, which is an indication that it was very tight and likely causing the headache. I put her in the "Slacken the Shoulder" position (see Appendix E) and immediately the sore spot in her upper trap muscle felt about 90% better. I held it there for two minutes. When I took her out of that position and touched the spot on her shoulder, the pain was 100% gone. She exclaimed that it felt like a miracle had just happened. "No miracle," I said. "Just good science."

Another big factor with headaches is lack of water. Even if your body is down just 1% of normal levels, the decline could trigger a headache.

I asked her if she was well hydrated and she said, "Yes, as a matter of fact I am drinking all day long."

"Good," I said. "What are you drinking?"

"I drink between 6–8 cups of coffee a day."

She didn't realize that coffee is a diuretic and actually takes water out of the body and dehydrates it. Caffeine also makes your muscles tighter. It can really give you a headache. I explained to her that the tight muscles in her shoulder and the lack of water in the tissues were more than likely the main causes of her headaches. I explained that it can take 6-8 weeks to rehydrate the tissues, so it was imperative that she cut back on the coffee to no more than two cups a day and start drinking a lot of water. Avoiding coffee altogether would be even better.

I put her on the Wellness Plan described above. I explained that this protocol usually works very well but that she would have to be consistent. Since pain is the great motivator, I was confident she would follow my instructions.

I saw her again about three months after that appointment. She reported that her headaches were mostly gone, occurring only now and then and usually when she had too much coffee. She also reported the side effects of feeling happier and having better memory recall.

This Wellness Plan has worked for many hundreds of my clients who suffer from headaches.

Temperomandibular Joint Disorder – TMJ

TMJ is the common abbreviation for Temporomandibular Joint Disorder. The temporomandibular joint, sometimes called the "jaw joint," is in front of the ear. The joint attaches the lower jaw to the skull and allows you to open and close your mouth, chew and speak. If this joint does not function properly, it can be very painful.

If you place two fingers on your jaw in front of the ear and chew, you can feel the joint moving. TMJ is a condition where tight muscles are putting pressure on the joint and in more severe cases even pulling it out of joint.

Tight muscles, or muscle imbalances in the neck, face and jaw muscles often start with a crooked pelvis because the spine is sitting on the pelvis. If the pelvis is crooked the spine is crooked. This means the tight muscles are either too long or too short and are pulling or compressing other structures in this area which can lead to the pain.

It is estimated that 10 million Americans suffer from TMJ. You can have tight, sore jaw muscles and not have TMJ. The protocol for getting rid of a tight jaw is the same as for TMJ. A tight jaw is often a precursor to TMJ.

You can improve or eliminate your TMJ or tight jaw with a little awareness and some self-care. It is vital to first identify and correct the common everyday activities that are causing muscle strain in the neck and shoulders that can lead to TMJ. There are many activities you do every day that may lead to pain and spasm either in the muscles of the jaw or those of the head, neck or shoulders.

We all have demands that keep us working through our pain. So we continually re-strain the area through our daily activities until we learn how to do those activities without causing muscle strain. The protocols listed in this book will help you perform your daily activities with little or no pain or show you how to relieve the pain that occurs because of these activities. Our plan is to reduce or eliminate as many causes of muscle strain as we can and apply stretches or slackenings to correct the muscle imbalances.

One of the most common causes of these muscle imbalances is simply poor posture and/or improper ergonomics. Slumping at your desk or in your car pushes your head forward of your body, putting a lot of strain on your neck and shoulders, which now have to hold up your head without the support of the spinal column. This strain can lead to TMJ. The average head weighs between 8-12 pounds. That is very heavy. If you tried to hold that much weight with your arms, you probably would not last more than five minutes. Yet we ask our neck and shoulder muscles to hold that weight all day long. These muscles are not designed to hold up your head. They are meant to move your head in different directions, not hold it in the same position for long periods of time. By correcting your computer and driving positions, you will bring your head over your shoulders, giving yourself good posture. Your bones (the spinal column) will be holding up your head, which will help take the strain off the muscles.

It is also very important to stretch the neck muscles every day. Many people have a head-forward posture, which will put quite a strain on the neck. A tight neck can lead to TMJ. Many people walk into my office rubbing their neck and saying that they hold all their stress in their neck. While this is true, it is not the kind of stress most people think. It is not so much "I got a ticket," "the boss yelled at me," or "the car broke down." This kind of emotional stress can of course add to the tension and pain in the neck muscles. The real source, however, is mostly a mechanical stress of having the head and/or arms forward of the body when either sitting or standing. Bad posture is responsible for a great amount of the stress in the neck.

By adopting the Wellness Plan in this chapter, you can eliminate or significantly reduce your TMJ pain. If after practicing the Wellness Plan you still have no improvement, see your health care provider for further assessment.

Symptoms:

TMJ is felt as pain in the jaw joint and/or the surrounding area. It may also be felt as ear pain and/or ringing in the ears. When the joint moves, you may hear sounds, such as clicking and/or popping. Other symptoms include swelling of the face or mouth, headache and dizziness. Your bite may feel uncomfortable. The jaw may also become locked in either the open or closed position.

Common Causes:

There are many lifestyle habits that can contribute to TMJ. The following are some of the most common I have come across in my practice.

- ◆ Tight muscles around the jaw (especially the masseter), grinding teeth and stress. This kind of stress makes your tight muscles even tighter. Try the breathing exercise described in Chapter 2.

- ◆ Chewing gum, poor posture, reading in bed, cradling a phone between your ear and shoulder and playing a wind or string instrument. These activities put a lot of strain on the neck, shoulder and jaw muscles that can lead to TMJ.

With a little awareness and by following the Wellness Plan in this book, you can easily make the changes in your life that will help stop your TMJ from returning.

Conventional Medical Approach

Standard medical treatments for TMJ often include pain-killers, muscle relaxants, cortisone shots or Botox injections. If these are not successful, surgery or corrective dental treatments are prescribed. Remember that the drugs and surgery do not always cure TMJ; rather, they hide the symptoms for a while. They are not addressing one of the biggest factors of TMJ — muscle imbalances.

IPT WELLNESS PLAN FOR TEMPOROMANDIBULAR JOINT DISORDER (TMJ)

MUSCLE REBALANCING: This section provides the exercises you need to do to correct the muscle imbalances that are causing your pain. By doing these exercises now, and continuing to do them as instructed, you will make your short muscles longer and your long muscles shorter and bring them back into balance.

Three Stretches to Balance the Pelvis (Appendix B)

These stretches will help to bring the body structure back into balance, thus eliminating a major cause of aches and pains. These exercises are designed to stretch the muscles or muscle groups that are typically too short in most people and are pulling the pelvis out of alignment. When the pelvis is crooked, it affects all the areas of the body. A pelvis that is out of alignment is often a cause of TMJ and headaches. Do these stretches twice a day.

Three Neck Stretches (Appendix C)

These stretches will loosen the muscles in the neck and shoulders and allow more blood and oxygen to flow to the head and neck. It takes about 90 seconds to do these stretches and doing them is a great habit to cultivate, as you will feel less pain and stiffness in the neck and you will be more alert. Consistent practice will reduce or eliminate a major cause of TMJ. Gently stretch the neck muscles three times a day.

Slacken the Jaw (Appendix D)

Slackening the jaw will help to loosen the masseter muscle in the jaw, which is usually very tight and short in most people. This tight muscle can refer pain to the head and/or pull the jaw out of alignment which can then lead to TMJ. Do this five times a day until the symptoms subside. Do not perform this exercise if it worsens the pain.

Slacken the Shoulders (Levator scapula & upper trapezius) (Appendix E)

Slackening the shoulders will relieve tension in the shoulders, especially the upper trap and levator scapula muscle. These tight muscles can contribute to TMJ. These areas are tight and sore in most people. Do this exercise any time you feel any tension in your shoulders or neck and at least five times a day. Do not do this exercise if it hurts to put your arm on top of your head.

Shoulder Shrugs (Appendix E)

Shoulder shrugs will help relax your shoulder and neck muscles and bring more blood and oxygen to the area, which will reduce tensions and pain. This will also help you feel more alert. Repeat several times throughout the day.

Strengthen Rhomboids (Appendix E)

Strengthening the rhomboids will help to shorten and strengthen the muscles between the shoulder blades, thus training the muscles to bring the head over the shoulders, improving the posture and reducing the strain on the neck and jaw. Do this ten times, three times a day.

Stretch the Chest (Pectoralis Major & Minor) (Appendix F)

In most people the chest muscles are too short and the rhomboids between the shoulder blades are too long, which give a person a head-forward, bent-over look with rounded shoulders. Stretching the chest muscles will release tension between the shoulder blades and open up the chest, which will make a person stand up straighter. When a person stands straight, the bones in the cervical spine hold up the head and the neck and jaw muscles can relax. Hold for at least 2 minutes. Do this exercise twice a day.

Slacken the Chest (Appendix F)

Slackening the chest muscles will relax the muscles in the chest, especially the pectoralis minor muscle. Relaxing these muscles helps people with shoulders rounded forward to bring them back into better alignment and will help to bring the head over the shoulder, thus reducing strain on the neck and jaw. Totally relax and hold that position for 2 minutes. Do this twice a day.

SUPPORTIVE LIFESTYLE: This part of your Wellness Plan is designed to address the root of the problem and to relieve habitual muscle imbalances to avoid aggravating the condition as you go about your daily life.

Check Sitting, Driving And Computer Positions (Appendix A)

Correcting your posture while sitting, driving and working at a computer will ensure the pelvis stays in balance and that you are not causing more stress on the neck, jaw, shoulders and lower and upper back. These common activities are responsible for a great amount of the pain in your life. Doing these activities the wrong way will make your body crooked and lead to muscle imbalances and possible lumbar or cervical disc problems. By slightly changing the way you perform these activities, you will keep the body in alignment and help ensure that once the pain is relieved it does not come back. Remember if you do what you always did, you get what you always got.

Keep Elbows Close To Body When Performing Daily Activities

Holding the arms away from the body for long periods can lead to tight sore muscles in many areas of your body like the jaw, neck and shoulders. In addition to your driving and computer positions, other common activities that cause muscle strain are using the phone and household activities like chopping vegetables or vacuuming. Performing your daily activities with your elbows close by your side will eliminate or prevent a lot of your pain.

Do Not Chew Gum

Chewing gum can tighten the muscles in the jaw and worsen the condition.

Slow Deep Breathing For 10-15 Minutes (see page 6)

Slow deep breathing relaxes the nervous system and thus relaxes the muscles in the jaw. Done just before bedtime, this exercise will help to reduce grinding of the teeth at night, which is a major cause of TMJ. Do this at least twice a day.

Success Story

This is the story of a 45-year-old male who had a stressful job and was suffering with jaw pain that was diagnosed as TMJ. He was using a bite plate that his dentist recommended and his doctor was recommending surgery. His pain levels were 5 on a scale of 10. He had been experiencing these symptoms for about a year. The pain was mostly in the jaw and the jaw made a clicking noise when opening and closing.

When I touched the masseter muscle, which is the big muscle in the jaw area, it was very painful with light pressure. I slackened the jaw and pressed the tissue again and he said that there was no pain at all. It was gone. I held that position for about two minutes and he said that he felt much better.

I still wanted to know what was giving him these muscle imbalances in the jaw and causing the pain. The cause is usually poor computer or driving positions. When I asked him to describe his office setup, it appeared to be a pretty good ergonomic setup. Upon further inquiry, I found out that he liked to read in bed at night propped up against the headboard with his head very forward. This position can cause a lot of pain in the neck, face or jaw.

I explained the Wellness Plan above to him and told him he needed to be consistent to get the results he wanted. His jaw pain went away almost immediately and he adopted the Wellness Plan, which kept the condition from coming back.

I have not only used this protocol to help many of my clients, but I also got rid of my own TMJ from many years of playing the trumpet.

7

Cervical Muscle Strain (Neck Pain)

The neck or cervical spine is that part of the body that connects the head to the trunk. It is comprised of muscles, nerves, arteries, bones and discs. These discs act like shock absorbers between the cervical vertebrae.

Neck pain can occur due to muscular tightness in both the neck and upper back or as a result of compressed nerves in this region. Almost everybody will experience a tight sore neck in his or her lifetime. In my 25 years of experience, I have only worked with a handful of people who did not have a tight neck.

Pain felt in the neck is usually caused by muscle imbalances in the neck, shoulder or upper back. This means the tight muscles are either too long or too short and are pulling or compressing other structures in this area, which can lead to the pain. A crooked pelvis is a contributor to neck pain because the spine sits on the pelvis.

You can improve or eliminate your neck pain with a little awareness and some self-care. It is vital to first identify and correct the common everyday activities that are causing muscle strain in the neck, shoulders or upper back that can lead to neck pain. Many activities you do every day may lead to pain and spasm in the muscles of the neck or shoulders or upper back.

We all have demands that keep us working through our pain. So we continually re-strain the area through our daily activities until we learn how to do those activities without causing muscle strain. The protocols listed in this book will help you perform your daily activities with little or no pain or show you how to relieve the pain that occurs because of these activities. Our plan is to reduce or eliminate as many causes of muscle strain as we can and apply stretches or slackenings to correct the muscle imbalances.

One of the most common causes of these muscle imbalances is simply poor posture and/or improper ergonomics. Slumping at your desk or in your car pushes your head forward of your body, putting a lot of strain on your neck and shoulders, which now have to hold up your head without the support of the spinal column. The average head weighs between 8–12 pounds. That is very heavy. If you tried to hold that much weight with your arms, you probably would not last more than 5 minutes. Yet we ask our neck and shoulder muscles to hold that weight all day long. These muscles are not designed to hold up your head. They are meant to move your head in different directions, not hold it in the same position for long periods of time. By correcting your computer and driving positions, you will bring your head over your shoulders, giving yourself good posture. Your bones (the spinal column) will be holding up your head, which will help take the strain off the neck muscles.

Lack of water can also be a factor in neck pain. In my opinion, many people do not drink enough water to adequately hydrate their cells. Muscles that do not get enough water ache more than muscles that are well hydrated. Also the discs need to be well hydrated to maintain their softness and avoid pinching or irritating a nerve. Good disc health is dependent on adequate water.

Remember that caffeine and alcohol are diuretics, which means they take water out of the body. It is fine to have these things in moderation, but remember to drink even more water. People will overlook the basics like drinking water and it is often the cause of many aches and pains. In general, drink half your body weight in ounces every day. Adequate fluid intake will help reduce the frequency of your neck pain and lead to better overall health. It can take up to six weeks to rehydrate, so please be patient. See Chapter 2 for more information about proper hydration.

It is also very important to stretch the neck muscles every day. Many people have a head-forward posture, which will put quite a strain on the neck. Many people walk into my office rubbing their neck and saying that they hold all their stress in their neck. While this is true, it is not the kind of stress most people think. It is not so much "I got a ticket," "the boss yelled at me," or "the car broke down." This kind of emotional stress can of course add to the tension and pain in the neck. The real source, however, is mostly a mechanical stress of having the head and/or arms forward of the body when either sitting or standing. Bad posture is responsible for a great amount of the pain and stress in the neck.

By adopting the Wellness Plan in this chapter, you can eliminate or significantly reduce your neck pain. If after practicing the Wellness Plan you still have no improvement, see your health care provider for further assessment.

Symptoms:

Pain in the neck could be described as an ache, tightness, burning or stabbing. This condition can be acute or chronic. It is often better or worse in certain positions such as lying down, sitting or standing. It can also radiate to other parts of the body such as down the arms or the upper back or head.

Common Causes:

There are many lifestyle habits that can contribute to neck pain. The following are some of the most common I have come across in my practice.

• Improper sitting positions, driving positions, standing positions and computer positions lead to head forward posture that can cause cervical muscle strain and perhaps lead to a disc problem.

• Emotional stress can also aggravate cervical muscle strain. Try the breathing exercise described in Chapter 2.

With a little awareness and by following the Wellness Plan in this book, you can easily make the changes in your life that will help stop your neck pain from returning.

Conventional Medical Approach

Standard medical treatments for neck pain often include pain-killers and muscle relaxants. Surgery is sometimes prescribed for nerve compression or herniated discs. Remember that the drugs and surgery do not always cure neck pain; rather they hide the symptoms for a while. They are not addressing one of the biggest factors of neck pain – muscle imbalances.

IPT WELLNESS PLAN FOR CERVICAL MUSCLE STRAIN (NECK PAIN)

MUSCLE REBALANCING: This section provides the exercises you need to do to correct the muscle imbalances that are causing your pain. By doing these exercises now, and continuing to do them as instructed, you will make your short muscles longer and your long muscles shorter and bring them back into balance.

Three Stretches to Balance the Pelvis (Appendix B)

These stretches will help to bring the body structure back into balance, thus eliminating a major cause of aches and pains. These exercises are designed to stretch the muscles or muscle groups that are typically too short in most people and are pulling the pelvis out of alignment. When the pelvis is crooked, this affects all the areas of the body. A pelvis that is out of alignment is often a major cause of neck strain and thus headaches, as many headaches are caused by tight neck muscles. Do these stretches twice a day.

Three Neck Stretches (Appendix C)

These stretches will loosen the muscles in the neck and shoulders and allow more blood and oxygen to flow to the head and neck. It takes about 90 seconds to do these stretches and doing them is a great habit to cultivate, as you will feel less pain and stiffness in the neck and you will be more alert. Consistent practice will reduce or eliminate the cause of a great amount of your neck pain. Gently stretch the neck muscles three times a day.

Slacken the Shoulders (Levator scapula & upper trapezius) (Appendix E)

Slackening the shoulders will relieve tension in the shoulders and neck, especially the upper trap and levator scapula muscle. These areas are tight and sore in most people. Do this exercise any time you feel any tension in your shoulders or neck and at least five times a day. Do not do this exercise if it hurts to put your arm on top of your head.

Shoulder Shrugs (Appendix E)

Shoulder shrugs will help relax your shoulder and neck muscles and bring more blood and oxygen to the area, which will reduce tension and pain. This will also help you feel more alert. Repeat several times throughout the day.

Strengthen Rhomboids (Appendix E)

Strengthening the rhomboids will help to shorten and strengthen the muscles between the shoulder blades, thus training the muscles to bring the head over the shoulders, improving the posture and reducing the strain on the neck. Do this ten times, three times a day.

Stretch the Chest (Pectoralis Major & Minor) (Appendix F)

In most people the chest muscles are too short and the rhomboids between the shoulder blades are too long, which give a person a head-forward, bent-over look with rounded shoulders. Stretching the chest muscles will release tension between the shoulder blades and open up the chest, which will make a person stand up straighter. When a person stands straight, the bones in the cervical spine hold up the head and the neck muscles can relax. Hold for at least two minutes. Do this exercise twice a day.

Slacken the Chest (Appendix F)

Slackening the chest muscles will relax the muscles in the chest, especially the pectoralis minor muscle. Relaxing these muscles helps people with shoulders rounded forward to bring them back into better alignment and will help to bring the head over the shoulder, thus reducing strain on the neck. Totally relax and hold that position for two minutes. Do this twice a day.

SUPPORTIVE LIFESTYLE: This part of your Wellness Plan is designed to address the root of the problem and to relieve habitual muscle imbalances to avoid aggravating the condition as you go about your daily life.

Check Sitting, Driving And Computer Positions (Appendix A)

Correcting your posture while sitting, driving and working at a computer will ensure the pelvis stays in balance and that you are not causing more stress on the neck, shoulders and lower and upper back. These common activities are responsible for a great amount of the pain in your life. Doing these activities the wrong way will make your body crooked and lead to muscle imbalances and possible lumbar or cervical disc problems. By slightly changing the way you perform these activities, you will keep the body in alignment and help ensure that once the pain is relieved it does not come back. Remember if you do what you always did, you get what you always got.

Walk or Stand Holding Your Wrist Behind Your Back

This stance will ensure that you have good posture when you are standing or walking. It will bring the head over the shoulders which will reduce or prevent neck pain. This will also open the chest and correct any pelvic tilt. This position should be used when you are walking slowly or standing in one place. When walking briskly, swing your arms naturally, which will help to move and clean out your lymphatic system, which is the body's sewer system.

Keep Elbows Close to Body When Performing Daily Activities

Holding the arms away from the body for long periods can lead to tight sore muscles in many areas of your body like the neck. In addition to your driving and computer positions, other common activities that cause muscle strain are using the phone and household activities like chopping vegetables or vacuuming. Performing your daily activities with your elbows close by your side will eliminate or prevent a lot of your pain.

Keep The Neck as Warm as Possible

Wear a collar, turtleneck shirt or scarf around your neck, even inside the house. Keeping the neck as warm as possible will help keep the neck loose and reduce the pain. A cold breeze on the neck is a factor in many headaches and stiff necks.

Heat Shoulders And Neck for 20 Minutes

Use a heating pad on the neck and shoulders every day for about 20 minutes. Applying warmth will help to relax the muscles in the area and bring more blood and oxygen to the tissues. Continue until the symptoms subside.

Keep Well Hydrated

Dehydration is a factor in cervical neck strain. Even slight dehydration can cause the neck muscles to ache. Many people are dehydrated. See Chapter 2 for instructions on how to drink water and how much. It can take up to six weeks to rehydrate.

Regular Exercise

Light regular exercise such as walking every day for at least 20 minutes can help with your neck pain by increasing your circulation. Exercise also releases certain neurotransmitters in the brain that can help eliminate pain.

Success Story

A woman in her 50s came to me complaining of a pain in the neck, which she has had for 20 years following a car accident. She was diagnosed with whiplash. The pain was in the back of the neck on the left side. Her pain was about a 6 on a scale of 10 and would often wake her at night. She had seen specialists all over the country and in Europe. Despite their best efforts, her pain remained. I had her point to where exactly she felt the pain. I performed the "slacken the shoulder" move and then very gently did the three neck stretches. When I asked her how her neck felt now, she had a surprised look on her face. She admitted that she had not thought I would be able to help her, but the pain in her neck was gone. She was actually a little bit angry. She said, "You mean I suffered for 20 years and this is all somebody needed to do?" She was sure that it was going to come back, so I explained the Wellness Plan to her and the importance of being diligent. I also explained how the pain resulting from whiplash is basically due to muscle imbalances. Once you know which muscles are too long and tight and which muscles are short and tight, it becomes quite easy to reduce or eliminate pain.

Almost every client I see has at least a tight neck if not a painful one. The above Wellness Plan only takes a few minutes a day and is a great practice for everyone to adopt.

8

Thoracic Outlet Syndrome (TOS)

The thoracic outlet is the space between the collarbone and the first rib. Thoracic Outlet Syndrome (TOS) is a compression of the nerves and/or blood vessels that affects the brachial plexus (nerves that pass into the arms from the neck) and various nerves and blood vessels in that space. This compression is due to muscle imbalances in the neck, chest, back and pelvis when not due to the presence of an extra rib called a cervical rib Tight muscles are either too long or too short and are pulling or compressing other structures in this area which can lead to the pain in the arms or hand.

You can improve or eliminate TOS with a little awareness and some self-care. It is vital to first identify and correct the common everyday activities that are causing muscle strain in the neck and shoulders that can lead to TOS. There are many activities you do every day that may lead to pain and spasm in the muscles of the head, neck, shoulders and back.

We all have demands that keep us working through our pain. So we continually re-strain the area through our daily activities until we learn how to do those activities without causing muscle strain. The protocols listed in this book will help you perform your daily activities with little or no pain or show you how to relieve the pain that occurs because of these activities. Our plan is to reduce or eliminate as many causes of muscle strain as we can and apply stretches or slackenings to correct the muscle imbalances.

One of the most common causes of these muscle imbalances is simply poor posture and/or improper ergonomics. Slumping at your desk or in your car pushes your head forward of your body, putting a lot of strain on your neck and shoulders, which now have to hold up your head without the support of the spinal column.

The average head weighs between 8 and 12 pounds. That is very heavy. If you tried to hold that much weight with your arms, you probably would not last more than 5 minutes. Yet we ask our neck and shoulder muscles to hold that weight all day long. These muscles are not designed to hold up your head. They are meant to move your head in different directions, not hold it in the same position for long periods of time.

By correcting your computer and driving positions, you will bring your head over your shoulders, giving yourself good posture. Your bones (the spinal column) will be holding up your head, which will help take the strain off the muscles. Holding your arms out on the steering wheel at the 10:00 and 2:00 positions is a major factor in TOS in my opinion. Bringing your arms down to the 4:00 and 8:00 positions will help take the strain off some of the muscles that are responsible for causing TOS.

It is also very important to stretch the neck muscles every day. This is especially true of the muscles on the side of the neck (scalenes). These muscles attach on the first rib. When tight, they pull up that rib, decreasing the space in the thoracic outlet and possibly causing compression of the nerves and blood vessels, which causes pain and tingling down the arm. Many people have a head-forward posture that causes quite a strain on the neck. A tight neck can lead to pain, fatigue and discomfort and possibly TOS. Many people walk into my office rubbing their neck and saying that they hold all their stress in their neck. While this is true, it is not the kind of stress most people think. It is not so much "I got a ticket," "the boss yelled at me," or "the car broke down." This kind of emotional stress can of course add to the tension and pain in the neck. The real source, however, is mostly a mechanical stress of having the head and/or arms forward of the body when either sitting or standing. Bad posture is responsible for a great amount of the mechanical stress in the neck.

It is also important to stretch and slacken the chest muscles. A tight, short pectoralis minor muscle in the chest can bring on numbness and tingling down the arm.

By adopting the Wellness Plan in this chapter, you can eliminate or significantly reduce your TOS. If after practicing the Wellness Plan you still have no improvement, see your health care provider for further assessment.

Symptoms:

Thoracic Outlet Syndrome is a sensation of pain, numbness, tingling, weakness, burning or coldness in the arm and/or hand caused by pressure on the nerves and/or blood vessels in the thoracic outlet. It can occur on one side of the body or both. The pain can be in the whole hand or just part of the hand, as in just the 4th and 5th fingers.

Tingling, pain or numbness indicates a compression of the nerves. Coldness indicates a compression of the blood vessels.

The symptoms of TOS are often confused with carpal tunnel, as they are similar. By performing the tests in Chapter 3, you will most often be able to tell which condition you have. Some people will have both conditions at the same time.

Common Causes:

There are many lifestyle habits that can contribute to thoracic outlet syndrome. The following are some of the most common I have come across in my practice.

- Repetitive activities that require the arms to be held over the head or outstretched
- Poor posture, especially head forward
- Improper computer and driving positions
- Cradling phone between shoulder and ear or holding phone to ear
- Riding a bike
- Whiplash
- Gardening

These activities can all cause muscle imbalances in the neck, shoulders and pelvis, which can cause compression of the brachial plexus in the thoracic outlet.

With a little awareness and by following the Wellness Plan in this book, you can easily make the changes in your life that will stop your pain from returning.

Conventional Medical Approach

Standard medical treatments for thoracic outlet syndrome often include pain-killers and muscle relaxants. Physical therapy is also widely prescribed for this condition. Surgery is sometimes prescribed for nerve compression or blood vessel constriction. Remember that drugs and surgery do not cure Thoracic Outlet Syndrome unless it is caused by the extra rib, called a "cervical rib." Rather, drugs and surgery hide the symptoms for a while. They are not addressing the biggest cause of TOS — muscle imbalances.

IPT WELLNESS PLAN FOR THORACIC OUTLET SYNDROME (TOS)

MUSCLE REBALANCING: This section provides the exercises you need to do to correct the muscle imbalances that are causing your pain. By doing these exercises now, and continuing to do them as instructed, you will make your short muscles longer and your long muscles shorter and bring them back into balance.

Three Stretches to Balance the Pelvis (Appendix B)

These stretches will help to bring the body structure back into balance, thus eliminating a major cause of aches and pains. These exercises are designed to stretch the muscles or muscle groups that are typically too short in most people and are pulling the pelvis out of alignment. When the pelvis is crooked, this affects all the areas of the body. A pelvis that is out of alignment is often a major cause of neck strain which can lead to Thoracic Outlet Syndrome. Do these stretches twice a day.

Three Neck Stretches (Appendix C)

These stretches will loosen the muscles in the neck and shoulders and allow more blood and oxygen to flow to the head and brain, reducing pain in the neck and head. It is especially important for relief of TOS to stretch the scalenes, which are the muscles on the side of the neck. Stretching the scalenes creates more space in the thoracic outlet, taking pressure off the nerves. Gently stretch the neck muscles three times a day.

Slacken the Shoulders (Levator scapula & upper trapezius) (Appendix E)

Slackening the shoulders will relieve tension in the shoulders, especially the upper trap and levator scapula muscle. These areas are tight and sore in most people. Do this exercise any time you feel any tension in your shoulders or neck and at least five times a day. Do not do this exercise if it hurts to put your arm on top of your head. This move might bring on some tingling which is okay for short periods of time.

Shoulder Shrugs (Appendix E)

Shoulder shrugs will help relax your shoulder and neck muscles and bring more blood and oxygen to the area, which will reduce tension and pain. This will also help you feel more alert. This exercise will create more space in your thoracic outlet and take pressure off the nerves, which is causing the symptoms. Repeat several times throughout the day.

Strengthen Rhomboids (Appendix E)

Strengthening the rhomboids will help to shorten and strengthen the muscles between the shoulder blades, thus training the muscles to bring the head over the shoulders, improving your posture, reducing strain on your neck and creating more space in the thoracic outlet. Do this ten times, three times a day.

Stretch the Chest (Pectoralis Major & Minor) (Appendix F)

In most people the chest muscles are too short and the rhomboids between the shoulder blades are too long, which give a person a head-forward, bent-over look with rounded shoulders. Stretching the chest muscles will release tension between the shoulder blades and open up the chest, which will make a person stand up straighter. When a person stands straight, the bones in the cervical spine hold up the head and the neck muscles can relax and there will be more space in the thoracic outlet. Hold for at least 2 minutes. Do this exercise twice a day.

Slacken the Chest (Appendix F)

Slackening the chest muscles will relax the muscles in the chest, especially the pectoralis minor muscle. Relaxing these muscles helps people with shoulders rounded forward to bring them back into better alignment and will help to bring the head over the shoulder, thus reducing strain on the neck and taking strain off the nerves in the thoracic outlet. Totally relax and hold that position for 2 minutes. Do this exercise twice a day.

SUPPORTIVE LIFESTYLE: This part of your Wellness Plan is designed to address the root of the problem and to relieve habitual muscle imbalances to avoid aggravating the condition as you go about your daily life.

Check Sitting, Driving and Computer Positions (Appendix A)

Correcting your posture while sitting, driving and working at a computer will ensure the pelvis stays in balance and that you are not causing more stress on the neck, shoulders and lower and upper back that can lead to TOS. These common activities are responsible for a great amount of the pain in your life. Doing these activities the wrong way will make your body crooked and lead to muscle imbalances and possible lumbar or cervical disc problems. By slightly changing the way you perform these activities, you will keep the body in alignment and ensure that once the pain is relieved it does not come back. Remember if you do what you always did, you get what you always got.

Walk or Stand Holding Your Wrist Behind Your Back

This stance will ensure that you have good posture when you are standing or walking. It will bring the head over the shoulders, open the chest and correct any pelvic tilt. This position should be used when you are walking slowly or standing in one place. When walking briskly, swing your arms naturally, which will help to move and clean out your lymphatic system, which is the body's sewer system.

Keep Elbows Close To Body When Performing Daily Activities

Holding the arms away from the body for long periods can lead to tight sore muscles in many areas of your body. In addition to your driving and computer positions, other common activities that cause muscle strain are using the phone and household activities like chopping vegetables or vacuuming. Performing your daily activities with your elbows close by your side will eliminate or prevent a lot of the symptoms of TOS.

Heat Your Shoulders and Thoracic Outlet Area

Put a heating pad on your shoulders and upper chest for 20 minutes. Do this every day until your symptoms subside.

Success Story

A woman in her 20s came to me suffering from numbness and tingling in her right hand and arm. She had been diagnosed with Thoracic Outlet Syndrome. She had had these symptoms for about six months. Although she was not in much pain, the numbness and tingling made it difficult for her to do her work as a massage therapist.

First I wanted to make sure that she really did have TOS, as carpal tunnel symptoms are very similar. I had her raise both hands over her head and wiggle her fingers. This is the test for TOS. Sure enough, in about 20 seconds, she started to have numbness and tingling.

The thoracic outlet is the space between the first rib and the collarbone. Symptoms develop when there is not enough space. The first thing I did was to see if her pelvis was crooked. It was elevated about 1.5 inches. Since the spine sits on the pelvis, the spine is also crooked. Since the ribs attach to the spine, the ribs become crooked, reducing the space in the thoracic outlet.

I did the three stretches to balance the pelvis, the three neck stretches and the Slacken the Chest move. I had her repeat the test for TOS by raising her hands over her head. No tingling this time.

The movements I did on her corrected her muscle imbalances and opened up the space in the thoracic outlet, preventing further nerve compression.

I explained the Wellness Plan listed above and told her it was very important to practice this every day so that her symptoms did not return.

9

Epicondylitis (Lateral and Medial)
(Tennis or Golfer's Elbow)

Lateral epicondylitis is inflammation and pain at the site of the lateral epicondyle where the wrist extensor muscles attach, by way of a tendon, to the little bony bump on the outside of the elbow. This condition is often called tennis elbow.

Medial epicondylitis is inflammation and pain at the site of the medial epicondyle where the wrist flexor muscles attach, by way of a tendon, to the little bony bump on the inside of the elbow. This condition is often called golfer's elbow.

Muscle imbalances in the forearm muscles mean the tight muscles are either too long or too short and are pulling or compressing other structures in this area, which leads to the elbow pain.

You can improve or eliminate epicondylitis with a little awareness and some self-care. It is vital to first identify and correct the common everyday activities that are causing muscle strain in the forearms that can lead to epicondylitis. There are many activities you do every day that may lead to pain and spasm in the muscles of the forearms.

We all have demands that keep us working through our pain. So we continually re-strain the area through our daily activities until we learn how to do those activities without causing muscle strain. The protocols listed in this book will help you perform your daily activities with little or no pain or show you how to relieve the pain that occurs because of these activities. Our plan is to reduce or eliminate as many causes of muscle strain as we can and apply stretches or slackenings to correct the muscle imbalances.

With tennis or golfer's elbow, the muscles and tendons that are involved are used in almost every daily activity – everything from brushing your teeth to typing at your computer. Basically, it affects any activity that involves using your hands. Proper posture and ergonomics will certainly help, but these tendons are in constant use throughout the day. It is very important to keep your wrist straight and unbent in all daily activities. A bent wrist in either direction puts strain on the elbow tendons and aggravates epicondylitis. If you have trouble keeping your wrist straight, use a wrist brace, which can be bought at any pharmacy, to help keep the wrist straight until the symptoms subside.

It is also very important to slacken these tendons every day by performing the Stretch and Slacken the Forearms exercise as described in the Wellness Plan. This will take the strain off of the tendon so it can begin to heal.

Lack of water can also be a factor in epicondylitis. In my opinion, many people do not drink enough water to adequately hydrate their cells. Muscles that do not get enough water ache more than muscles that are well hydrated. Also, the elbow joint needs to be well hydrated to maintain good lubrication. Good joint health is dependent on adequate water.

Remember that caffeine and alcohol are diuretics, which means they take water out of the body. It is fine to have these things in moderation, but remember to drink even more water. People will overlook the basics like drinking water and it is often the cause of many aches and pains. In general, drink half your body weight in ounces every day. Fluid intake will help reduce the frequency of your pain and lead to better overall health. It can take up to six weeks to rehydrate, so please be patient. See Chapter 2 for more information on proper hydration.

Do not rest your arms on the armrest of a chair. Resting your arms on armrests can interfere with the motion of the forearm muscles as they contract and relax, which can aggravate epicondylitis.

Rest is still one of nature's best healing methods. Since tennis or golfer's elbow is usually an overuse injury, resting your arms and hands, or a least reducing the amount of activity, will speed up the healing process.

By adopting the Wellness Plan in this chapter, you can eliminate or significantly reduce epicondylitis. If after practicing the Wellness Plan you still have no improvement, see your health care provider for further assessment.

Symptoms:

Pain or stiffness at the site of the elbow sometimes radiating to other parts of the arm. The pain is often worse when typing or squeezing objects. The pain usually occurs in the dominant arm, although in can be in the other arm or both arms.

Common Causes:

Many lifestyle habits can contribute to tennis or golfer's elbow. The following are some of the most common I have come across in my practice.

- Working at a computer
- Playing a musical instrument
- Knitting

- ◆ Cutting vegetables
- ◆ Carpentry
- ◆ Tennis
- ◆ Golf
- ◆ Painting
- ◆ Lifting heavy objects
- ◆ Gripping objects too firmly

These activities can all cause muscle imbalances in the forearm muscles that attach to the elbow. Limiting these activities when you have a sore elbow will speed up the recovery process.

With a little awareness and by following the Wellness Plan in this book, you can easily make the changes in your life that will help stop your elbow pain from returning.

Conventional Medical Approach

Standard medical treatments for tennis or golfer's elbow often include pain-killers, muscle relaxants and anti-inflammatory drugs. Physical therapy is also widely prescribed for this condition. Surgery is sometimes prescribed to clean up damaged tissue. Remember that drugs and surgery do not always cure epicondylitis; rather they hide the symptoms for a while. They are not addressing one of the biggest factors of epicondylitis – muscle imbalances.

IPT Wellness Plan for Epicondylitis (Lateral and Medial) (Tennis or Golfer's Elbow)

MUSCLE REBALANCING: This section provides the exercises you need to do to correct the muscle imbalances that are causing your pain. By doing these exercises now, and continuing to do them as instructed, you will make your short muscles longer and your long muscles shorter and bring them back into balance.

Slacken the Thumb (Hand squeeze) (Appendix G)

Slackening the thumb will release the muscle in the thumb called pollicis and the other muscles on the palm side of the hand. Although it is not the primary muscle involved in epicondylitis this muscle is usually tight and sore as well. Hold for two minutes. Do this as many times through out the day as you can.

Elbow Tendon Release (Appendix G)

Releasing the elbow tendons will take strain off the muscles in the forearm that can contribute to epicondylitis. Hold for two minutes. Do this five times a day.

Slacken and Stretch the Forearm (Wrist flexors and extensors) (Appendix G)

Slackening and stretching the forearm muscles will release the tight muscles that can contribute to epicondylitis. These tight muscles will pull on the elbow and may bring on symptoms. Hold each position for two minutes. Do this ten times a day, reducing the number of repetitions as the pain subsides. If one of the directions causes pain, only do the one that feels good.

SUPPORTIVE LIFESTYLE: This part of your Wellness Plan is designed to address the root of the problem and to relieve habitual muscle imbalances to avoid aggravating the condition as you go about your daily life.

Check Sitting, Driving and Computer Positions (Appendix A)

Correcting your posture while sitting, driving and working at a computer will ensure the pelvis stays in balance and that you are not causing more stress on the neck, shoulders and lower and upper back by holding your arms and hands in positions that can indirectly bring on the symptoms of epicondylitis. These common activities are responsible for a great amount of the pain in your life. Doing these activities the wrong way will make your body crooked and lead to muscle imbalances and possible lumbar or cervical disc problems. By slightly changing the way you perform these activities, you will keep the body in alignment and help ensure that once the pain is relieved it does not come back. Remember if you do what you always did, you get what you always got.

Keep Elbows Close To Body When Performing Daily Activities

Holding the arms away from the body for long periods can lead to tight sore muscles in many areas of your body. In addition to your driving and computer positions, other common activities that cause muscle strain are using the phone and household activities like chopping vegetables or vacuuming. Performing your daily activities with your elbows close by your side will eliminate or prevent a lot of your pain. Do not rest your arms on the armrests of a chair, as this can aggravate epicondylitis.

Keep Your Wrist Straight In All Daily Activities

For activities that you must do during the day, keep your wrist straight. A bent wrist puts pressure on the elbow tendons and can bring on symptoms. If it is difficult to keep a straight wrist, use a wrist brace for this purpose. Try to be aware of your wrist position so that you don't become dependent on the brace. Use it as a short-term tool during recovery and to help you learn proper wrist position.

Rest Your Arms

Activities involving your hands are the main cause of this condition. Limiting or avoiding using your hands for a while in conjunction with the other exercises listed here will help alleviate the pain.

Heat Forearms for 20 Minutes

Use a heating pad on your forearms every day for about 20 minutes. Continue until your symptoms subside.

Ice Your Elbow

If there is a lot of pain in the elbow, icing it for about 10 minutes will often bring quick relief. You can ice your elbow at the same time as you heat the forearm.

Success Story

A man in his 40s came to see me with a diagnosis from his doctor of tennis elbow (lateral epicondylitis). He had been suffering with this condition for about a year. His job involved sitting at a computer all day and in fact he was also a tennis player. More people today get tennis elbow from their computer than actually do from tennis. Both these activities can cause tennis elbow.

This condition is sometimes hard to clear up because we have to use the muscles in the forearm a lot in our daily activities, thus re-injuring the elbow every day.

When I touched the tissue at the site of the elbow, it was very sore. I performed the move to slacken and stretch the forearm. I touched the tissue again and the pain was gone for the first time in a year.

I explained to him that although the pain was gone, the inflammation was still there and he could easily re-injure those muscles. I advised him to give up tennis for 4 weeks and showed him how to slacken the forearm muscles. I had him do this slackening ten times a day for two minutes each time for about two weeks. Then he was to reduce the frequency to about five times a day for maintenance.

I saw him two months later and he reported that as long as he did the Wellness Plan his pain did not return. If he stopped following the plan, the pain would start to creep back.

As a massage therapist, I use my hands a lot and it would be easy to get tennis elbow. I slacken my forearms five times a day to keep myself pain-free.

10

Carpal Tunnel Syndrome (CTS)

The carpal tunnel is a small space located on the palm side of the wrist. It is formed on the bottom by the wrist bones and on the top by the retinaculum, which is a band of connective tissue. The median nerve and several tendons that help bend your fingers run through this space – like going through a tunnel. Carpal Tunnel Syndrome (CTS) is a condition in which the median nerve is compressed at the wrist in the tunnel. Bending the wrist decreases the size of the tunnel. The median nerve is the only nerve that runs through the tunnel. The pain associated with CTS is often due to muscle imbalances in the forearm muscles. The tight muscles in the forearm are either too long or too short and are pulling or compressing other structures in this area, especially the median nerve, which leads to the pain or numbness.

You can improve or eliminate CTS with a little awareness and some self-care. It is vital to first identify and correct the common everyday activities that are causing muscle strain in the arms and hands that can lead to CTS. We all have demands that keep us working through our pain. So we continually re-strain the area through our daily activities until we learn how to do those activities without causing muscle strain. The protocols listed in this book will help you perform your daily activities with little or no pain or show you how to relieve the pain that occurs because of these activities. Our plan is to reduce or eliminate as many causes of muscle strain as we can and apply stretches or slackenings to correct the muscle imbalances.

With Carpal Tunnel Syndrome, the muscles and tendons that are involved are used in almost every daily activity – everything from brushing your teeth to typing at your computer. It is aggravated by any activity that involves using your hands. Proper posture and ergonomics will certainly help, but these tendons and muscles are in constant use throughout the day. It is very important to keep your wrist straight and unbent in all daily activities. A bent wrist in either direction puts strain on the median nerve, aggravating CTS. If you have trouble keeping your wrist straight, use a wrist brace, which can be bought at any pharmacy, to help keep the wrist from bending until the symptoms subside. It is especially important to wear the wrist brace at night, as many people sleep with a bent wrist, which can bring on the symptoms.

It is also very important to slacken the area of the carpal tunnel every day. This will often take the strain off of the median nerve so it can begin to heal. In the beginning, you should do this about ten times a day. You can decrease that number as your symptoms subside.

Also have your health care provider check your vitamin B-12 levels. Low levels of B-12 are associated with Carpal Tunnel Syndrome.

Lack of water can also be a factor in CTS. In my opinion, many people do not drink enough water to adequately hydrate their cells. Muscles that do not get enough water ache more than muscles that are well hydrated. Also the joints need to be well hydrated to maintain their lubrication. Good joint health is dependent on adequate water.

Remember that caffeine and alcohol are diuretics, which means they take water out of the body. It is fine to have these things in moderation, but remember to drink even more water. People will overlook the basics like drinking water and it is often the cause of many aches and pains. In general, drink half your body weight in ounces every day. Adequate fluid intake will help reduce the pain associated with CTS and lead to better overall health. It can take up to six weeks to rehydrate, so please be patient. See Chapter 2 for more information on proper hydration.

Do not rest your arms on the armrest of a chair. Resting your arms on armrests can interfere with the motion of the forearm muscles and tendons as they contract and relax. This position can aggravate Carpal Tunnel Syndrome.

Rest is still one of nature's best healing methods. Since CTS is usually an overuse injury, resting your arms and hands, or a least reducing the amount of activity, will speed up the healing process.

Soaking the area in Epsom salt and warm water will often bring relief.

By adopting the Wellness Plan in this chapter, you can eliminate or significantly reduce CTS. If after practicing the Wellness Plan you still have no improvement, see your health care provider for further assessment.

Symptoms:

Carpal Tunnel Syndrome is a sensation of pain, numbness, tingling, burning or weakness in the hand and fingers caused by pressure on the median nerve in the carpal tunnel. This condition especially affects the thumb and the first two fingers. It is often accompanied by loss of grip strength, making it hard to hold a cup or phone. It is sometimes accompanied by swelling of the hand.

Common Causes:

There are many lifestyle habits that can contribute to Carpal Tunnel Syndrome. The following are some of the most common I have come across in my practice.

- Sitting at a computer
- Playing a musical instrument
- Knitting
- Cutting vegetables
- Carpentry
- Sleeping with bent wrists
- Painting
- Lifting heavy objects
- Gripping objects too firmly
- Biking

These activities can all cause muscle imbalances in the forearm muscles, which affects the carpal tunnel. Limiting these activities when you have Carpal Tunnel Syndrome will speed up the recovery process.

Conventional Medical Approach

Standard medical treatments for Carpal Tunnel Syndrome often include pain killers, muscle relaxants and anti-inflammatory drugs. Physical therapy is also widely prescribed for this condition. Surgery is sometimes prescribed to take the pressure off the median nerve, which is causing the pain and numbness. Remember that drugs and surgery do not always cure CTS; rather they hide the symptoms for a while. They are not addressing one of the biggest factors of CTS – muscle imbalances.

IPT WELLNESS PLAN FOR CARPAL TUNNEL SYNDROME (CTS)

MUSCLE REBALANCING: This section provides the exercises you need to do to correct the muscle imbalances that are causing your pain. By doing these exercises now, and continuing to do them as instructed, you will make your short muscles longer and your long muscles shorter and bring them back into balance.

Slacken the Thumb (Hand Squeeze) (Appendix G)

Slackening the thumb will release the muscle in the thumb called pollicis and the other muscles on the palm side of the hand. This will also create more space in the carpal tunnel, taking pressure off the median nerve. Hold for 2 minutes. Do this exercise as many times throughout the day as you can.

Slacken and Stretch the Forearm (wrist flexors and extensors) (Appendix G)

Slackening and stretching the forearm muscles will release the tight forearm that can contribute to CTS. Tight forearm muscles may decrease the space in the carpal tunnel and bring on symptoms. Hold each position for two minutes. Do this ten times a day, reducing the number of repetitions as the pain subsides. If one of the directions causes pain only do the one that feels good.

SUPPORTIVE LIFESTYLE: This part of your Wellness Plan is designed to address the root of the problem and to relieve habitual muscle imbalances to avoid aggravating the condition as you go about your daily life.

Check Sitting, Driving and Computer Positions (Appendix A)

Correcting your posture while sitting, driving and working at a computer will ensure the pelvis stays in balance and that you are not causing more stress on the neck, shoulders and lower and upper back that can indirectly lead to Carpal Tunnel Syndrome by holding your arms and hands in positions that can bring on the symptoms. These common activities are responsible for a great amount of the pain in your life. Doing these activities the wrong way will make your body crooked and lead to muscle imbalances and possible lumbar or cervical disc problems. By slightly changing the way you perform these activities, you will keep the body in alignment and help ensure that once the pain is relieved it does not come back. Remember if you do what you always did, you get what you always got.

Rest Arms and Hands

Cut back on your daily activities as much as possible until your symptoms are improved. Typing, knitting, playing an instrument and chopping vegetables are typical activities that make your forearm muscles tight and bring on symptoms. Rest is still nature's great healer.

Keep Your Wrist Straight In All Daily Activities

For activities that you must do during the day, keep your wrist straight. A bent wrist puts pressure on the median nerve and will bring on symptoms. If it is difficult to keep a straight wrist, use a wrist brace for this purpose. Try to be aware of your wrist position so that you don't become dependent on the brace. Use it as a short term tool during recovery and to help you learn proper wrist position.

Wear a Wrist Brace At Night To Keep Your Wrist Straight

Carpal tunnel is often worse at night because most people sleep with a bent wrist. This position will put pressure on the median nerve all night. Wearing a wrist brace at night will help.

Heat Forearm and Hands

Use a heating pad on your hands, wrists and forearms. Do this once or twice a day for at least 20 minutes. Continue until your symptoms subside.

Check Vitamin B-12 levels

Have your health care provider check your B-12 levels. Low levels of B-12 are associated with Carpal Tunnel Syndrome.

Soak Hands and Wrists in Epsom Salt

Soak your hands and wrists in a little tub of warm water for about 20 minutes a night for five nights. Make the water deep enough to cover your wrists. Use about one pound of Epsom salt to three to five gallons of water. Epsom salt is magnesium sulphate. It is a natural muscle relaxant and a natural anti-inflammatory.

Success Story

A woman in her 20s came to see me with a diagnosis of Carpal Tunnel Syndrome. She'd had these symptoms for about six months and her doctor had recommended surgery. She worked at a desk job at the computer all day. Upon further inquiry, I found out she was also a knitter. Both of these activities can lead to Carpal Tunnel Syndrome.

CTS is often hard to clear up as the muscles involved are used often in our everyday life. I recommended she give up knitting for at least a month and that she wear a wrist brace to keep her wrist straight. A bent wrist will keep aggravating the median nerve. I told her to wear it while sleeping and during the day.

I showed her how to slacken the thumb, which will often relieve the symptoms of CTS. When I tried to do slacken the forearm muscles, both directions were painful, so of course we did not pursue that exercise.

I told her to heat her forearm muscles every night for about 20 minutes.

I also explained the importance of drinking enough water to keep the hand and wrist well lubricated.

She later reported to me that the symptoms of her carpal tunnel started to get a little better in about four days and have continued to improve. She is hopeful now that she will not need the surgery.

11

Lumbar Muscle Strain
(Low Back Pain)

The lower back is a large area that connects the upper body to the lower body. Pain felt in the lower back is usually caused by muscle imbalances in this lumbar region. The tight muscles are either too long or too short and are pulling or compressing other structures in this area which leads to the pain. Tight muscles will often pull the pelvis out of alignment and/or cause the spine to be crooked and/or aggravate a disc problem. Pain may also radiate from other areas like the mid or upper back.

Low back pain is very common. Almost every one will experience low back pain at some time in their life. It is estimated that we spend $50 billion each year on this condition. Headache and low back pain are the two most common reasons people seek medical attention.

You can improve or eliminate low back pain with a little awareness and some self-care. It is vital to first identify and correct the common everyday activities that are causing muscle strain that can lead to low back pain. There are many activities you do every day that may lead to pain in the muscles of the head, neck, shoulders or back.

We all have demands that keep us working through our pain. So we continually re-strain the area through our daily activities until we learn how to do those activities without causing muscle strain. The protocols listed in this book will help you perform your daily activities with little or no pain or show you how to relieve the pain that occurs because of these activities. Our plan is to reduce or eliminate as many causes of muscle strain as we can and apply stretches or slackenings to correct the muscle imbalances.

One of the most common causes of these muscle imbalances is simply poor posture and/or improper ergonomics. Slumping at your desk or in your car pushes your head forward of your body and rounds out the lower back. This puts a lot of strain on your neck, shoulders and low back, which will likely pull the pelvis out of alignment. Keeping your back rounded for long periods of time in your chair is a major factor in low back pain. I believe that half the back pain in the country could be eliminated if everyone sat with the proper support. By correcting your computer and driving positions, you will bring your head over your shoulders and straighten out your back, giving yourself good posture. Your bones (the spinal column) will be doing their job, which will help take the strain off the muscles.

Pelvic misalignment is very common and often causes low back pain. There are three common ways the pelvis is misaligned: 1) it is higher on one side; 2) it is rotated; 3) it is tilted either forward or backward. Most people have at least one of these imbalances and many have all three. The stretches described in the Wellness Plan for Lumbar Muscle Strain will help realign the pelvis.

Lack of water can also be a factor in low back pain. In my opinion, many people do not drink enough water to adequately hydrate their cells. Muscles that do not get enough water ache more than muscles that are well hydrated. Also, the discs need to be well hydrated to maintain their softness and avoid pinching or irritating a nerve. Discs should be about 80% water. Good disc health is dependent on adequate water. As an interesting note, in a recent study it was found that 70% of herniated discs cause no pain in the body.

Remember that caffeine and alcohol are diuretics, which means they take water out of the body. It is fine to have these things in moderation, but remember to drink even more water. People will overlook the basics like drinking water and it is often the cause of many aches and pains. In general, drink half your body weight in ounces every day. Fluid intake will help reduce the frequency of your low back pain and lead to better overall health. It can take up to six weeks to rehydrate, so please be patient. See Chapter 2 for more information on proper hydration.

By adopting the Wellness Plan in this chapter, you can eliminate or significantly reduce your back pain. If after practicing the Wellness Plan you still have no improvement, see your health care provider for further assessment.

Symptoms:

Pain in the low back that could be described as an ache, tightness, burning or stabbing. This condition can be acute or chronic. It is often better in certain positions such as lying down, standing or sitting. It may be painful to get up out of a chair or bed. The pain may also radiate down the legs. This is often accompanied by pain in the groin.

Common Causes:

There are many lifestyle habits that can contribute to low back pain. The following are some of the most common I have come across in my practice.

- Long periods of improper standing
- Long periods of improper sitting
- Sports – especially one-sided sports like tennis and golf
- Lifting heavy objects

These activities can all cause muscle imbalances in the low back (lumbar region), which can lead to low back pain. Limiting these activities when you have lumbar muscle strain will speed up the recovery process.

The following conditions are caused by muscle imbalances and are a major source of low back pain.

+ Unbalanced pelvis
+ Tight, short quadriceps
+ Externally rotated legs
+ Some disc problems

Conventional Medical Approach

Standard medical treatments for low back pain often include pain-killers, muscle relaxants, anti-depressants, cortisone and anti-inflammatory drugs. Physical therapy is also widely prescribed for this condition. Surgery is sometimes prescribed if other measures are not working. Remember that drugs and surgery do not always cure low back pain; rather they hide the symptoms for a while. They are not addressing the biggest cause of lumbar muscle strain – muscle imbalances.

IPT WELLNESS PLAN FOR LUMBAR MUSCLE STRAIN (LOW BACK PAIN)

MUSCLE REBALANCING: This section provides the exercises you need to do to correct the muscle imbalances that are causing your pain. By doing these exercises now, and continuing to do them as instructed, you will make your short muscles longer and your long muscles shorter and bring them back into balance.

Three Stretches to Balance the Pelvis (Appendix B)

These stretches will help to bring the body structure back into balance, thus eliminating a major cause of aches and pains. These exercises are designed to stretch the muscles or muscle groups that are typically too short in most people and are pulling the pelvis out of alignment. When the pelvis is crooked, all areas of the body are affected. A pelvis that is out of alignment is often a major cause of neck strain and low back pain because those muscles are out of balance. Do these stretches twice a day.

Slacken the Hip Flexors (Psoas and Quadriceps) (Appendix H)

The hip flexor muscles are typically too short in most people. The very act of sitting in a chair, which we have done our entire lives, makes the hip flexors short. These short hip flexors will pull the pelvis forward resulting in an anterior pelvic tilt which can cause an exaggerated curve in the low back and low back pain or disc problems. This is a very common problem. Slackening the hip flexors relaxes these muscles and lets the pelvis release back to neutral, which can alleviate pain. Do this exercise three or more times a day for two minutes or longer each time.

Half-Frog (Slacken the Piriformis) (Appendix H)

The half-frog position will slacken the piriformas muscle and take strain off the low back and the sacro-illiac joint on either side of your low back. Hold for two minutes or more. Repeat on the other side. Do this five or more times a day, reducing the repetitions as your symptoms start to subside. If this position hurts on one side, only do the side that feels good.

Slacken the Inside of the Thigh (adductors) (Appendix I)

Most people sit with their legs and feet turned out to the sides. Sitting with your legs and feet slightly turned in will slacken the inside thigh muscles (adductors) and take strain off the lower back and the knees. Do not walk or stand in this position. Do this only when you are sitting. Do this every time you sit.

Strengthen the Inside of the Thigh (adductors) (Appendix I)

Strengthening the adductor muscles will shorten the muscles on the inside of the upper leg and pull the legs back into alignment in a neutral position so that the strain is taken off the low back and the knees. Do ten of these compressions and then rest for a minute and do ten more. Continue in this manner until you can do about five sets of ten. This exercise will strengthen the muscles on the inside of your legs and begin to reduce your symptoms.

SUPPORTIVE LIFESTYLE: This part of your Wellness Plan is designed to address the root of the problem and to relieve habitual muscle imbalances to avoid aggravating the condition as you go about your daily life.

Check Sitting, Driving and Computer Positions (Appendix A)

Correcting your posture while sitting, driving and working at a computer will ensure the pelvis stays in balance and that you are not causing more stress on the neck, shoulders and lower and upper back. These common activities are responsible for a great amount of the pain in your life. Doing these activities the wrong way will make your body crooked and lead to muscle imbalances and possible lumbar or cervical disc problems. By slightly changing the way you perform these activities, you will keep the body in alignment and help ensure that once the pain is relieved it does not come back. Remember if you do what you always did, you get what you always got.

Heat Sore Areas for 20 minutes

Use a heating pad on the sore areas every day for about 20 minutes. Continue until the symptoms subside.

Success Story

This is the story of a man in his 40s who suffered severe back pain for almost two years. It was difficult for him to stand or sit for long periods, but there was little or no pain when lying down. His doctor did an MRI of the region and found nothing unusual. This man was sitting at a desk all day for his work.

Most low back pain is simply due to muscle imbalances in the pelvic region resulting in a crooked pelvis. Most people are crooked in three ways. This man certainly was when I measured him.

I performed three stretches to bring his pelvis back into balance and showed him how to do these stretches himself. I also showed him the proper sitting, computer and driving positions that would help keep his pelvis straight.

He was a little nervous about getting off my table, because that movement was usually very painful. Much to his surprise, there was only a little pain when getting off the table. He was already much improved.

I stressed to him the importance of the Wellness Plan so that his pain would not return. He could not believe how simple it was to bring him out of pain after two years of suffering.

12

Piriformis Syndrome – Sciatica

The sciatic nerve has several branches coming out of the spinal cord into the lower back. Parts of the nerve run through the buttocks and down the back of each leg to the ankle and foot. When the sciatic nerve is irritated or compressed by a disc or a tight muscle, there could be pain in the low back, buttocks or down the leg into the foot. This is generally called Sciatica. When this compression is caused by the piriformis muscle, it is called Piriformis Syndrome.

Piriformis syndrome and muscle related sciatica are caused by muscle imbalances in the hip and buttock muscles. Tight muscles are either too long or too short and are pulling or compressing other structures in this area, which leads to the pain. This condition is prevalent with people who sit improperly for long periods of time.

You can improve or eliminate muscle related sciatica and Piriformis Syndrome with a little awareness and some self-care. It is vital to first identify and correct the common everyday activities that are causing muscle strain that can lead to sciatica. There are many activities you do every day that may lead to pain and spasm in the muscles of the head, neck, shoulders or back.

We all have demands that keep us working through our pain. So we continually re-strain the area through our daily activities until we learn how to do those activities without causing muscle strain. The protocols listed in this book will help you perform your daily activities with little or no pain or show you how to relieve the pain that occurs because of these activities. Our plan is to reduce or eliminate as many causes of muscle strain as we can and apply stretches or slackenings to correct the muscle imbalances.

One of the most common causes of these muscle imbalances is simply poor posture and/or improper ergonomics. Slumping at your desk or in your car pushes your head forward of your body and rounds out the lower back. This puts a lot of strain on your neck, shoulders and low back, which will likely pull the pelvis out of alignment. Keeping your back rounded for long periods of time in your chair is a major cause of sciatic compressions. I believe that half the back pain in the country could be eliminated if everyone sat with the proper support. By correcting your computer and driving positions, as described in the Wellness Plan, you will bring your head over your shoulders and straighten out your back, giving yourself good posture. Your bones (the spinal column) will be holding up your head, which will take the strain off the muscles.

It is very important that you perform the three stretches to balance the pelvis. These three stretches usually bring the pelvis back into alignment. There are three common ways the pelvis is misaligned. 1) It is higher on one side; 2) it is rotated; 3) it is tilted either forward or backward. Most people have at least one of these imbalances and many have all three. A balanced pelvis usually loosens the piriformis and takes the pressure off the sciatic nerve.

Although it is a common practice to stretch the piriformis, I have found that stretching this muscle will often aggravate sciatica. When you stretch a muscle, you temporarily make it tighter, like stretching a rubber band. This tightness then aggravates the nerve. Slackening usually feels very good by taking pressure off the nerve. See the Wellness Plan for instructions for Slackening the Piriformis, which often brings dramatic relief along with instructions for Slackening the Hip Flexors, another exercise which can bring quick relief from sciatic pain.

Lack of water can also be a factor in sciatic pain. In my opinion, many people do not drink enough water to adequately hydrate their cells. Muscles that do not get enough water ache more than muscles that are well hydrated. Also, the discs needs to be well hydrated to maintain their softness and prevent pinching or irritating a nerve. Discs should be about 80% water. Good disc health is dependent on adequate water.

Remember that caffeine and alcohol are diuretics, which means they take water out of the body. It is fine to have these things in moderation, but remember to drink even more water. People will overlook the basics like drinking water and it is often the cause of many aches and pains. In general, drink half your body weight in ounces every day. Fluid intake will help reduce the frequency of your sciatic pain and lead to better overall health. It can take up to six weeks to rehydrate, so please be patient. See Chapter 2 for more information on proper hydration.

By adopting the Wellness Plan in this chapter, you can eliminate or significantly reduce your sciatica. If after practicing the Wellness Plan you still have no improvement, see your health care provider for further assessment.

Symptoms:

Symptoms of Piriformis Syndrome or sciatica include pain that begins in your back or buttocks and moves down your leg and may move into your foot. Weakness, tingling, or numbness in the leg may also occur. These symptoms could indicate a disc problem or a tight piriformis. This condition is often worse when sitting or standing. Symptoms can range from mild to severe.

Common Causes:

There are many lifestyle habits that can contribute to sciatica. The following are some of the most common I have come across in my practice.

- Biking
- Sitting improperly
- Driving; especially a clutch

These activities can all cause muscle imbalances in the low back (lumbar region), which can lead to sciatica. Limiting these activities when you have sciatica will speed up the recovery process.

The following conditions caused by muscle imbalances are a major source of sciatica.

- Tight piriformis
- Disc problems

These two physiological changes can also cause sciatica:

- Spinal stenosis
- Pregnancy

Conventional Medical Approach

Standard medical treatments for sciatica pain often include pain killers, muscle relaxants, anti-depressants, cortisone and anti-inflammatories. Physical therapy is also widely prescribed for this condition. Surgery is sometimes prescribed if these other measures are not working. Remember that drugs and surgery do not cure sciatica unless it is due to spinal stenosis or other boney or disc impingement on the sciatic nerve which can be relieved surgically. Otherwise, drugs and surgery don't address one of the biggest factors of sciatica – muscle imbalances.

IPT WELLNESS PLAN FOR PIRIFORMIS SYNDROME (SCIATICA)

MUSCLE REBALANCING: This section provides the exercises you need to do to correct the muscle imbalances that are causing your pain. By doing these exercises now, and continuing to do them as instructed, you will make your short muscles longer and your long muscles shorter and bring them back into balance.

Three Stretches to Balance the Pelvis (Appendix B)

These stretches will help to bring the body structure back into balance, thus eliminating a major cause of aches and pains. These exercises are designed to stretch the muscles or muscle groups that are typically too short in most people and are pulling the pelvis out of alignment. When the pelvis is crooked, all the areas of the body are affected. A pelvis that is out of alignment is often a major cause of Piriformis Syndrome or sciatica. Do these stretches twice a day.

Half-Frog (Slacken the Piriformis) (Appendix H)

The Half-Frog position will slacken the piriformis muscle and take strain off the sciatic nerve. Hold for two minutes or more. Repeat on the other side. Do this five or more times a day and less frequently as your symptoms start to subside. If this hurts on one side, only do the side that feels good.

Slacken the Hip Flexors (Psoas and Quadriceps) (Appendix H)

The hip flexor muscles are typically too short in most people. The very act of sitting in a chair, which we have done our whole lives, makes the hip flexors short. These short hip flexors will pull the pelvis forward, resulting in an anterior pelvic tilt which can cause an exaggerated curve in the low back and/or sciatica or disc problems. This is a very common condition. Slackening the hip flexors relaxes these muscles, allows the pelvis to return to neutral and relieves pain.

Slacken the Inside of the Thigh (Adductors) (Appendix I)

Most people sit with their legs and feet turned out to the sides. Sitting with your legs and feet slightly turned in will slacken the adductors, gently release the piriformis and take strain off the lower back and knees. Do not walk or stand like this. Do this only when you are sitting.

Strengthen the Inside Thighs (Adductors) (Appendix I)

Strengthening the adductor muscles will shorten the muscles on the inside of the upper leg and pull the legs back into neutral alignment so that the strain is taken off the low back and the knees and the piriformis can release. Do ten of these compressions and then rest for a minute and do ten more. Continue in this manner until you can do about five sets of ten. This exercise will strengthen the muscles on the inside of your legs and begin to reduce your symptoms.

SUPPORTIVE LIFESTYLE: This part of your Wellness Plan is designed to address the root of the problem and to relieve habitual muscle imbalances to avoid aggravating the condition as you go about your daily life.

Check Sitting, Driving and Computer Positions (Appendix A)

Correcting your posture while sitting, driving and working at a computer will ensure the pelvis stays in balance and that you are not causing more stress on the neck, shoulders and lower and upper back that can compress the sciatic nerve that can lead to sciatica or Piriformis Syndrome.

These common activities are responsible for a great amount of the pain in your life. Doing these activities the wrong way will make your body crooked and lead to muscle imbalances and possible lumbar or cervical disc problems. By slightly changing the way you perform these activities, you will keep the body in alignment and help ensure that once the pain is relieved it does not come back. Remember if you do what you always did, you get what you always got.

Use Heat on Low Back and Buttocks

Use a heating pad on your low back and buttocks every day for about 20 minutes. Continue until your symptoms subside.

Success Story

This is the story of a man in his 50s suffering from sciatica. The pain was in his left buttock and traveling down the back of the left leg as well. He had this pain on and off for about 10 years. He had been to physical therapy many times with only moderate relief. His doctor had given up on him.

It is almost always what you are doing every day that gives you your aches and pains. I wanted to know what he did for a living. He said he was a truck driver. I asked him if his truck had a clutch. He said it did and admitted that his pain was always worse when driving. I have seen this many times before. People usually have their foot on the clutch with the foot turned out, which in turn contracts the piriformis even more. In this man's case, this position was really compressing the sciatic nerve, which was sending the pain down his leg.

First I had him do the three stretches to balance the pelvis, which was quite crooked. Then I had him lie face down. I pressed on his piriformis gently. It was so tight and inflamed that he jumped and gave out a yelp. I immediately put him into the position known as half-frog, which will slacken the piriformis. I gently pressed the piriformis again. He said that the pain was gone. I pressed the piriformis a little harder and still he said there was no pain in the half-frog position.

I explained to him that it was crucial that he adapt the correct sitting and driving positions and that he needed to keep his foot on the clutch straight and not turned out. Before he got off my table, I told him there would be some pain still because the nerve was irritated and inflamed. I advised him that if he followed the Wellness Plan as described in this chapter, his pain would more than likely be all gone in about two weeks.

He came to see me about a month later and indeed his pain was gone. He remained pain-free as long as he used the proper lumbar support and kept his foot straight when using the clutch.

I encouraged him to keep performing the Wellness Plan, even though he felt better, so that his sciatica would not return.

13

Knee Pain and Medial Meniscus

The medial meniscus is a band of cartilage on the inside of the knee at the head of the tibia. There is also one on the outside of the knee. It is a common site of injury, especially in sports. The medial meniscus acts as a shock absorber between the tibia and the femur. Large tears to the meniscus may require surgery. Small tears will respond well to the protocols in this book. The meniscus is often damaged due to muscle imbalances in the hip and leg muscles. The tight muscles are either too long or too short and are pulling or compressing the meniscus and other structures in this area, which leads to the pain.

Knee replacements have almost doubled in the last ten years. The truth is that your knees should last longer than you do. They will not wear out as long as your pelvis is straight and there is no underlying problem like rheumatoid arthritis. Think of our car example. If the front end of your car is out of alignment, your tires will wear out quickly. In this case, your tires are your knees. Keep the pelvis straight to save your knees. A straight pelvis will allow your knees to take the stress on them the way nature intended and they will last a long time.

You can improve or eliminate your knee pain with a little awareness and some self-care. It is vital to first identify and correct the common everyday activities that are causing muscle strain in the pelvis and legs that can lead to pain in the knee. We all have demands that keep us working through our pain. So we continually re-strain the area through our daily activities until we learn how to do those activities without causing muscle strain. The protocols listed in this book will help you perform your daily activities with little or no pain or show you how to relieve the pain that occurs because of these activities. Our plan is to reduce or eliminate as many causes of muscle strain as we can and apply stretches or slackenings to correct the muscle imbalances.

One of the most common causes of these muscle imbalances is simply poor posture and/or improper ergonomics. Slumping at your desk or in your car pushes your head forward of your body and rounds out the lower back. This position puts a lot of strain on your neck, shoulders and low back, which will likely pull the pelvis out of alignment. Keeping your back rounded for long periods of time in your chair is a major cause of a crooked pelvis, which then leads to strain on the knees. I believe a great deal of the knee pain in the country could be eliminated if everyone sat with the proper support. By correcting your computer and driving positions, you will bring your head over your shoulders and straighten your back, giving yourself good posture. Your bones will be supporting you, which will take the strain off the muscles.

Many people walk and sit with their feet turned out, which puts a lot of strain on the knee, especially on the inside (medial). It is important to correct the muscle imbalances that lead to walking this way. We need to train the feet to go back to the neutral position, which is pointing straight ahead. Try to sit with your toes slightly turned in. This position will often quickly take the strain off the knee and relieve the pain. Do not stand or walk with your toes turned in. Just sit that way.

When the feet are turned out, the muscles on the outside of the leg are too short. Doing the stretch we call Abductor Stretch will lengthen those muscles and start to bring the feet straighter, which will often take the strain off the knee.

Knee pain is also often caused by your quadriceps being too short. These are the muscles on the front of the upper leg. They attach at the knee. If they are too short, they can cause knee pain. Gently stretching these muscles will help to alleviate the pain.

Lack of water can also be a factor in knee pain. In my opinion, many people do not drink enough water to adequately hydrate their cells. Muscles that do not get enough water ache more than muscles that are well hydrated. Also, the knee joint needs to be well hydrated in order to keep it well lubricated, which will reduce or eliminate any inflammation in the knee. Good joint health is dependent on adequate water.

Remember that caffeine and alcohol are diuretics, which means they take water out of the body. It is fine to have these things in moderation, but remember to drink even more water. People will overlook the basics like drinking water and it is often the cause of many aches and pains. In general, drink half your body weight in ounces every day. Fluid intake will help reduce the frequency of your knee pain and lead to better overall health. It can take up to six weeks to rehydrate, so please be patient. See Chapter 2 for more information about proper hydration.

By adopting the Wellness Plan in this chapter, you can eliminate or significantly reduce your knee pain. If after practicing the Wellness Plan you still have no improvement, see your health care provider for further assessment.

Symptoms:

Symptoms include pain on the inside of the knee, often accompanied by swelling. This can indicate anything from a sprain to a tear. The area is often painful to the touch. There may also be limited range of motion or popping and clicking sounds with movement. It is also often accompanied by pain in the groin.

Common Causes:

There are many lifestyle habits that can contribute to knee pain. The following are some of the most common I have come across in my practice.

- ◆ Sports
- ◆ Dancing
- ◆ Driving
- ◆ Yoga
- ◆ Weightlifting

These activities can all cause muscle imbalances in the knee, which can lead to knee or medial meniscus pain. Limiting these activities when you have knee pain will speed up the recovery process.

The following conditions caused by muscle imbalances are a major source of knee pain.

- ◆ Imbalanced pelvis
- ◆ External rotators of the leg too short

Conventional Medical Approach

Standard medical treatments for knee pain often include pain-killers, muscle relaxants, hyaluronic acid injections, cortisone and anti-inflammatories. Physical therapy is also widely prescribed for this condition. Surgery is sometimes prescribed if other measures are not working. Remember that drugs and surgery do not always cure knee pain; rather they hide the symptoms for a while. They are not getting to one of the biggest causes of knee pain — muscle imbalances.

IPT Wellness Plan for Medial Meniscus Injury (Knee Pain)

MUSCLE REBALANCING: This section provides the exercises you need to do to correct the muscle imbalances that are causing your pain. By doing these exercises now, and continuing to do them as instructed, you will make your short muscles longer and your long muscles shorter and bring them back into balance.

Three Stretches to Balance the Pelvis (Appendix B)

These stretches will help to bring the body structure back into balance, thus eliminating a major cause of aches and pains. These exercises are designed to stretch the muscles or muscle groups that are typically too short in most people and are pulling the pelvis out of alignment. When the pelvis is crooked, all the areas of the body are affected. A pelvis that is out of alignment is often a major cause of knee pain. Do these stretches twice a day.

Half-Frog (Slacken the Piriformis) (Appendix H)

The Half-Frog position will slacken the piriformis muscle allowing the leg and knee to return to a neutral position, taking strain off the knee. Hold the position for two minutes or more. Repeat on the other side. Do this five or more times a day and then less frequently as your symptoms start to subside. If this hurts on one side, only do the side that feels good.

Slacken the Hip Flexors (Psoas & Quadriceps) (Appendix H)

The hip flexor muscles are typically too short in most people. The very act of sitting in a chair, which we have done our whole lives, makes the hip flexors short. These short hip flexors will pull the pelvis forward resulting in an anterior pelvic tilt which can cause an exaggerated curve in the low back. Some of the hip flexors attach near the knee and can put a lot of strain on the knee, a common condition. Slackening the hip flexors relaxes these muscles, allows the pelvis to return to neutral and takes the strain off the knee.

Slacken the inside of the thigh (adductors). (Appendix I)

Most people sit with their legs and feet turned out to the sides. Sitting with your legs and feet slightly turned in will take strain off the lower back and the knees. Do not walk or stand in this position. Do it only when you are sitting.

Strengthen the Inside Thighs (After Some Healing Occurs) (adductors) (Appendix I)

After some healing occurs and your knee pain lessens you can strengthen the adductors. Strengthening the adductors will shorten the muscles on the inside of the upper leg and pull the legs back into neutral alignment so that strain is taken off the low back and the knees. Do ten of these compressions and then rest for a minute and do ten more. Continue in this manner until you can do about five sets of ten. This exercise will strengthen the muscles on the inside of your legs and begin to reduce your symptoms.

SUPPORTIVE LIFESTYLE: This part of your Wellness Plan is designed to address the root of the problem and to relieve habitual muscle imbalances to avoid aggravating the condition as you go about your daily life.

Check Sitting, Driving and Computer Positions (Appendix A)

Correcting your posture while sitting, driving and working at the computer will ensure the pelvis stays in balance and that you are not placing more stress on the knees. These common activities are responsible for a great amount of the pain in your life. Doing these activities the wrong way will make your body crooked. By slightly changing the way you perform these activities, you will keep the body in alignment and help make sure that once the pain is relieved it does not come back. Remember if you do what you always did, you get what you always got.

Use Heat on the Quadriceps

The quadriceps are the muscles on the front part of the upper leg. Use a heating pad to warm the quadriceps 20 minutes every night. This will help to loosen those muscles and take strain off the knees.

Success Story

A woman in her 60s who was an avid yoga practitioner came to me complaining of moderate to severe knee pain in both knees. She had already had an operation to repair a tear in the medial meniscus on her left side. Now her doctor was telling her that she would probably need an operation on the other knee as well. Her doctor gave her some pain medication and she was going to physical therapy, which she said was making it worse.

She complained that the inside of her thighs, especially around the knee and groin, felt very tight. She was doing a lot of yoga stretches for that area but she could not seem to get that tissue to feel loose no matter how much stretching she did.

I had her lie on her back and I observed that her feet turned way out almost like a ballet dancer. In this condition, the tissue on the outside of the thigh is too short and tight whereas the tissue on the inside of the thigh is too long and tight like an overstretched rubber band. I touched the inside of her knees and they were very sore. I turned her legs and feet in for two minutes to rebalance those muscles affecting the knees. When I touched the tissue again, there was no pain. She could not believe it, as her knees had been sore for years.

Once I explained to her how the tissue was too long on the inside of her thighs and that stretching that tissue was making it worse, she understood.

I advised her to stop all stretching for the inside of the thigh (known in yoga as "hip openers"). I showed her how to strengthen the adductors and sit with the feet turned in.

I showed her the three stretches to balance the pelvis and told her to do only those three stretches for about a month. She was not to stretch any other muscles.

Her knees recovered quickly and she did not need an operation on her other knee.

I stressed the importance of the Wellness Plan to make sure that her symptoms did not return.

14

Plantar Fasciitis – Heel Spur

Plantar fasciitis is inflammation of the plantar fascia. This is the tissue that forms the arch of the foot. Plantar means bottom of the foot. Fascia is connective tissue and -*itis* means inflammation.

A heel spur is a hook of bone that can form on the heel. Plantar fasciitis is often accompanied by a heel spur that can be seen on an x-ray. Heel spurs are soft, bendable deposits of calcium that are a result of mechanical tension and inflammation. Heel spurs do not cause pain. They are an indication that plantar fasciitis may be present, which is what is causing the pain.

This condition is often due to muscle imbalances in the pelvis, lower leg and foot muscles. The tight muscles are either too long or too short and are pulling or compressing other structures in this area, which often leads to the pain.

You can improve or eliminate your plantar fasciitis with a little awareness and some self-care. It is vital to first identify and correct the common everyday activities that are causing muscle strain in the pelvis, lower leg and foot muscles that can lead to plantar fasciitis. There are many activities you do every day that may lead to pain and inflammation in these muscles.

We all have demands that keep us working through our pain. So we continually re-strain the area through our daily activities until we learn how to do those activities without causing muscle strain. The protocols listed in this book will help you perform your daily activities with little or no pain or show you how to relieve the pain that occurs because of these activities. Our plan is to reduce or eliminate as many causes of muscle strain as we can and apply stretches or slackenings to correct the muscle imbalances.

One of the most common causes of these muscle imbalances is simply poor posture and/or improper ergonomics. Slumping at your desk or in your car pushes your head forward of your body and rounds out the lower back. This position puts a lot of strain on your neck, shoulders and low back, which will likely pull the pelvis out of alignment. Keeping your back rounded for long periods of time in your chair is a major cause of a crooked pelvis, which then leads to strain on the feet and possibly plantar fasciitis. By correcting your computer and driving positions, you will bring your head over your shoulders and straighten your back, giving yourself good posture. Your bones (spinal column) will be supporting you, which will help take the strain off the muscles.

Many people walk and sit with their feet turned out, which puts a lot of strain on the feet. It is important to correct the muscle imbalances that lead to walking this way. We need to train the feet to go back to the neutral position, which is pointing straight ahead. Try to sit with your toes slightly turned in. Do not stand or walk with your toes turned in. Just sit that way.

The standard medical treatment for plantar fasciitis is to stretch the calf and ice the foot. I have found that this method may take months or years to heal the condition. Far more effective is to slacken the calf and foot and heat the foot by soaking it in warm water and Epsom salt every night. This will often bring relief in weeks not months.

If you have plantar fasciitis, it is important to wear shoes with good arch supports. The arch support puts the bottom of the foot into slack and helps to relieve the pain. Walking barefoot or in flip-flops can aggravate plantar fasciitis.

Lack of water can also be a factor in plantar fasciitis. In my opinion, many people do not drink enough water to adequately hydrate their cells. Muscles that do not get enough water ache more than muscles that are well hydrated. Water is a good anti-inflammatory.

Remember that caffeine and alcohol are diuretics, which means they take water out of the body. It is fine to have these things in moderation, but remember to drink even more water. People will overlook the basics like drinking water and it is often the cause of many aches and pains. In general, drink half your body weight in ounces every day. Fluid intake will help reduce the frequency of your foot pain and lead to better overall health. It can take up to six weeks to rehydrate, so please be patient. See Chapter 2 for more information on proper hydration.

By adopting the Wellness Plan in this chapter, you can eliminate or significantly reduce your plantar fasciitis. If after practicing the Wellness Plan you still have no improvement, see your health care provider for further assessment.

Symptoms:

The most common complaint is pain in the bottom of the heel or other part of the plantar area. It is usually worse in the morning and improves throughout the day. It often occurs in conjunction with a tight, sore calf and/or Achilles tendon.

Common Causes:

There are many lifestyle habits that can contribute to plantar fasciitis. The following are some of the most common I have come across in my practice.

- Long periods of standing or walking
- Running
- Dancing
- Wearing improper shoes

These activities or habits can all cause muscle imbalances in the calf and foot, which can lead to plantar fasciitis. Limiting these activities when you have plantar fasciitis will speed up the recovery process. Wear shoes that have good arch supports.

The following conditions caused by muscle imbalances are a major source of plantar fasciitis.

- Imbalanced hip
- Tight calf
- Tight Achilles tendon
- Flat feet

Conventional Medical Approach

Standard medical treatments for plantar fasciitis often include pain-killers, muscle relaxants, cortisone and anti-inflammatories. Physical therapy is also widely prescribed for this condition. Orthotics and a night splint that keeps the calf stretched all night are common prescriptions. Surgery is sometimes prescribed if other measures are not working. Remember that drugs and surgery do not always cure plantar fasciitis; rather they hide the symptoms for a while. They are not addressing the biggest factor in plantar fasciitis – muscle imbalances.

IPT WELLNESS PLAN FOR PLANTAR FASCIITIS (HEEL SPUR)

MUSCLE REBALANCING: This section provides the exercises you need to do to correct the muscle imbalances that are causing your pain. By doing these exercises now, and continuing to do them as instructed, you will make your short muscles longer and your long muscles shorter and bring them back into balance.

Three Stretches to Balance the Pelvis (Appendix B)

These stretches will help to bring the body structure back into balance, thus eliminating a major cause of aches and pains. These exercises are designed to stretch the muscles or muscle groups that are typically too short in most people and are pulling the pelvis out of alignment. When the pelvis is crooked, this affects all the areas of the body. A pelvis that is out of alignment is often a major cause of plantar fasciitis. Do these stretches twice a day.

Achilles Tendon Release (Appendix J)

The Achilles tendon is the thick cord on the back of the heel that attaches the calf to the heel. Releasing this tendon takes the strain off the calf and the plantar area (bottom of the foot). Hold the position for two minutes and do the exercise three times a day.

Slacken the Calf (Appendix J)

Slackening the calf releases the calf muscle and the Achilles tendon and gives almost immediate relief. Hold the position for two minutes. Do this exercise at least five times a day. In this case the more often you slacken the calf the better.

Gentle Stretching of Calf Muscles (Appendix J)

Stretching the calf will lengthen the muscle and takes the strain off the bottom of the foot. Do not stretch too deeply. Stretching deeply can aggravate plantar fasciitis. If this hurts, the stretch is too deep. Do this 5–10 times a day and less frequently as the pain starts to subside.

Strengthen the Inside Thighs (Adductors) (Appendix I)

Strengthening the adductor muscles will shorten the muscles on the inside of the upper leg and pull the legs back into alignment so that strain is taken off the low back and the knees. When your legs are in their neutral position, your feet will strike the ground as nature intended when you are walking and this will help alleviate plantar fasciitis. Do ten of the compressions and then rest for a minute and do ten more. Continue in this manner until you can do about five sets of ten.

Slacken the Inside of the Thigh (adductors) (Appendix I)

Most people sit with their legs and feet turned out to the sides. Sitting with your legs and feet slightly turned in will train your body to walk with your feet straight and thus take strain off the plantar fascia. Do not walk or stand in this position. Do this only when you are sitting.

SUPPORTIVE LIFESTYLE: This part of your Wellness Plan is designed to address the root of the problem and to relieve habitual muscle imbalances to avoid aggravating the condition as you go about your daily life.

Sitting, Driving and Computer Positions (Appendix A)

Correcting your posture while sitting, driving and working at the computer will ensure the pelvis stays in balance and that you are not causing more stress on the plantar fascia and Achilles tendon. These common activities are responsible for a great amount of the pain in your life. Doing these activities the wrong way will make your body crooked. By slightly changing the way you perform these activities, you will keep the body in alignment and help make sure that once the pain is relieved it does not come back. Remember if you do what you always did, you get what you always got.

Proper Arch Support

Walking barefoot aggravates plantar fasciitis. Always wear shoes with good arch supports. Good arch supports keep the calf muscles and the bottom of the foot in slack. Fortunately, most of the brand names have good arch support. Athletic shoes are best. Avoid sandals and flip-flops until your pain goes away.

Rest

If you are a runner or are on your feet a lot, good old-fashioned rest will be quite helpful. Rest is still nature's great healer. The more you can rest, the more quickly you will see results.

Soak Your Feet in Epsom Salt and Warm Water

Soak your feet in a little tub of warm water for about 20 minutes a night for five nights. Make the water deep enough to cover your Achilles tendon. Use about 1 pound of Epsom salt to 3-5 gallons of water. Epsom salt is magnesium sulphate. It is a natural muscle relaxant and a natural anti-inflammatory.

Success Story

A man in his 30s came to me. He had been diagnosed with plantar fasciitis. X-rays showed he also had a heel spur. He had very sharp pain on the bottom of his heel when standing or walking. He had been a runner, but had not been able to run for the last 8 months because of the pain. His doctor had given him a cortisone shot, which helped for a couple of weeks. He was going to physical therapy, which was only helping a little. He was also wearing a boot at night that kept his calf and Achilles tendon stretched all night. He stated that the pain was about 8 on a scale of 10.

I have treated many cases of plantar fasciitis and I know that the standard medical approach seldom brings the desired results. I had him lie face down on my table and I pressed the spot on his heel where the pain was located. He reported that it was very painful. I put him in the "slacken the calf" position and pressed the spot again. He said it was still sore but much less so. I held that position for two minutes and then pressed the spot again. He said there was no pain. He couldn't believe it could be that easy!

He wanted to know if he could start running again.

I explained to him that although he felt better, he still had some inflammation and that the pain would return if he did not follow the Wellness Plan to rebalance his muscles. I told him that after he rebalanced his muscles and the inflammation died down, he could slowly start running again.

On a follow-up visit, he reported that he had started running about two weeks after he last saw me and had been running ever since. I encouraged him to continue to follow the Wellness Plan so that his symptoms would not return.

15

Fibromyalgia

Fibromyalgia means pain in the muscles, ligaments, and tendons — the soft tissues in the body. Fibromyalgia is a chronic condition with widespread pain in the muscles, ligaments and tendons, as well as fatigue and multiple tender points. Tender points can be found in the back of the neck, shoulders, chest, lower back, hips, elbows, and knees. The pain may spread from these areas. These tender points will be on both the left and right side of the body and both above and below the waist.

This condition is often due to muscle imbalances in many different muscles all over the body. Tight muscles are either too long or too short and are pulling or compressing other structures in the body, which leads to pain.

People with fibromyalgia tend to wake up with body aches and stiffness. This is often because they have not had any water all night. Fibromyalgia is more common in women than in men. Other names for this condition are fibrositis, chronic muscle pain syndrome, and tension myalgias. You can improve or eliminate your fibromyalgia with a little awareness and some self-care. It is vital to first identify and correct the common everyday activities that are causing muscle strain in the neck, shoulders, upper and lower back and arms and legs that can lead to fibromyalgia. There are many activities you do every day that may lead to widespread pain and spasm in the muscles in various parts of the body.

We all have demands that keep us working through our pain. So we continually re-strain the area through our daily activities until we learn how to do those activities without causing muscle strain. The protocols listed in this book will help you perform your daily activities with little or no pain or show you how to relieve the pain that occurs because of these activities. Our plan is to reduce or eliminate as many causes of muscle strain as we can and apply stretches or slackenings to correct the muscle imbalances.

One of the most common causes of these muscle imbalances is simply poor posture and/or improper ergonomics. Slumping at your desk or in your car pushes your head forward of your body and rounds out the lower back. This position puts a lot of strain on your neck, shoulders and low back, which will likely pull the pelvis out of alignment. Keeping your back rounded for long periods of time in your chair is a major cause of a crooked pelvis, which then leads to strain in widespread areas of the body which could be diagnosed as fibromyalgia. By correcting your computer and driving positions, you will bring your head over your shoulders and straighten your back, giving yourself good posture. Your bones (the spinal column) will be supporting you, which will take the strain off the muscles and reduce or eliminate the pain.

Lack of water can also be a factor in fibromyalgia. In my opinion, many people do not drink enough water to adequately hydrate their cells. Muscles that do not get enough water ache more than muscles that are well hydrated. Also, the discs need to be well hydrated to maintain their softness and avoid pinching or irritating a nerve. Good disc health is dependent on adequate water. I have observed that most of the people who come to me with a diagnosis of firbromyalgia are dehydrated to a greater or lesser degree.

Remember that caffeine and alcohol are diuretics, which means they take water out of the body. It is fine to drink them in moderation, but remember to drink even more water. If you have fibromyalgia, you may want to eliminate caffeine and alcohol completely until you start to feel better. People overlook the basics like drinking water and it is often the cause of many aches and pains. In general, drink half your body weight in ounces every day. Increased fluid intake will help to reduce the frequency of your pain and stiffness and lead to better overall health. It can take up to six weeks to rehydrate, so please be patient. See Chapter 2 for more information on proper hydration.

By adopting the Wellness Plan in this chapter, you can eliminate or significantly reduce your widespread pain. If after practicing the Wellness Plan you still have no improvement, see your health care provider for further assessment.

Symptoms:

There is chronic, widespread pain with tenderness to light touch. The pain can be mild to severe and is often accompanied by fatigue. There can also be tingling of the skin that feels like needles. There may also be nerve pain and brain fog. Trouble sleeping is common.

Common Causes:

There is no known cause of fibromyalgia, but the following are significant contributors:

- Postural deviations
- Improper sitting posture
- Improper driving positions
- Improper computer positions

These activities can all cause muscle imbalances in the body, which can lead to fibromyalgia. Limiting or correcting these activities will speed up the recovery process.

The following habits lead to chemical imbalances in the body, muscle pain and fatigue.

- Lack of water
- Too much caffeine
- Poor diet

Conventional Medical Approach

Standard medical treatments for fibromyalgia often include pain-killers, muscle relaxants, anti-depressants, anti-seizure drugs and anti-inflammatories. Remember that the drugs do not cure fibromyalgia; rather they hide the symptoms for a while. They are not addressing one of the biggest factors in fibromyalgia – muscle imbalances.

IPT WELLNESS PLAN FOR FIBROMYALGIA

MUSCLE REBALANCING: This section provides the exercises you need to do to correct the muscle imbalances that are causing your pain. By doing these exercises now, and continuing to do them as instructed, you will make your short muscles longer and your long muscles shorter and bring them back into balance.

Three Stretches to Balance the Pelvis (Appendix B)

These stretches will help to bring the body structure back into balance, thus eliminating a major cause of aches and pains. These exercises are designed to stretch the muscles or muscle groups that are typically too short in most people and are pulling the pelvis out of alignment. When the pelvis is crooked, all areas of the body are affected. A pelvis that is out of alignment is often a factor in fibromyalgia. Do these stretches twice a day.

Three Neck Stretches (Appendix C)

Gently stretch the neck muscles three times a day. Loosening the muscles in the neck and shoulders will allow more blood and oxygen to flow to the head and neck. It takes about 90 seconds to stretch these muscles. It is a great habit to cultivate, as you will feel less pain and stiffness in the neck and you will be more alert. Consistent practice will reduce or eliminate the cause of your neck pain and help with "brain fog."

Slacken the Shoulders (Levator scapula & upper trapezius) (Appendix E)

Slackening the shoulders will relieve tension in the shoulders especially the upper trap and levator scapula muscle. These areas are tight and sore in most people. Hold the position for at least two minutes. Do this exercise any time you feel any tension in your shoulders or neck and at least five times each day. Do not do this exercise if it hurts to put your arm on top of your head.

Stretch the Chest (Pectoralis Major & Minor) (Appendix F)

In most people the chest muscles are too short and the rhomboids between the shoulder blades are too long, which gives a person a head-forward, bent-over look with rounded shoulders. Stretching the chest muscle will release tension between the shoulder blades and open up the chest, which will make a person stand up straighter. When a person stands straight, the bones in the cervical spine support the head and the neck muscles can relax. Hold the positions for at least two minutes and do the exercise twice a day.

Slacken the Chest (Appendix F)

Slackening the chest will relax the muscles in the chest, especially the pectoralis minor muscle. Relaxing these muscles helps people with shoulders rounded forward to bring them back into better alignment and will help bring the head over the shoulder, reducing strain on the neck. Totally relax and hold the position for two minutes.

Slacken the Calf (Appendix J)

Slackening the calf releases the calf muscle and the Achilles tendon. Do this exercise at least five times a day. In this case, more often is better.

Gentle Stretching of Calf Muscles (Appendix J)

Stretching the calf will lengthen the muscle and relieve the pain in that area. Do not stretch too deeply. If this hurts, the stretch is too deep. Do this 5–10 times a day and then less frequently as the pain starts to subside.

Strengthen the Inside Thighs (adductors) (Appendix I)

Strengthening the adductor muscles will shorten the muscles on the inside of the upper leg and pull the legs back into neutral alignment so that the strain is taken off the low back and knees. Do ten of the compressions and then rest for a minute and do ten more. Continue in this manner until you can do about five sets of ten. This exercise will strengthen the muscles on the inside of your legs and begin to reduce your symptoms.

Slacken the Inside of the Thigh (adductors) (Appendix I)

Most people sit with their legs and feet turned out to the sides. Sitting with your legs and feet slightly turned in will take strain off the lower back and the knees. Do not walk or stand in this position. Do this only when you are sitting.

SUPPORTIVE LIFESTYLE: This part of your Wellness Plan is designed to address the root of the problem and to relieve habitual muscle imbalances to avoid aggravating the condition as you go about your daily life.

Check Sitting, Driving and Computer Positions (Appendix A)

Correcting your posture while sitting, driving and working at the computer will ensure the pelvis stays in balance and that you are not causing more stress on the neck, shoulders and lower and upper back that can lead to Fibromyalgia symptoms. These common activities are responsible for a great amount of the pain in your life. Doing these activities the wrong way will make your body crooked. By slightly changing the way you perform these activities, you will keep the body in alignment and ensure that once the pain is relieved it does not come back. Remember if you do what you always did, you get what you always got

Keep Well Hydrated

One of the most common causes of widespread pain is dehydration. Even slight dehydration can cause muscle ache and cramps. Many people are dehydrated. If you have fibromyalgia, start hydrating as soon as possible. See Chapter 2 for instructions on how to drink water and how much. It can take up to six weeks to rehydrate.

Epsom Salt Bath

Soak your body in a tub of warm water for about 20 minutes. Use about four pounds of Epsom salt every night for 5 nights. Epsom salt is magnesium sulphate. It is a natural muscle relaxant and a natural anti–inflammatory.

Heat Sore Areas for 20 Minutes

Use a heating pad on sore areas every day for about 20 minutes. The heat will help the muscles relax and feel better. Continue this treatment until the symptoms subside.

Success Story

A 30-year-old woman came to me with a diagnosis from her doctor of fibromyalgia. She was in constant pain. Her muscles and especially her joints were very sore. This pain was spread over most of her body. Depending on the day, her pain levels were anywhere between 6–8 on a scale of 10. She was having trouble remembering things and she was also experiencing depression. Her doctor had prescribed pain-killers and antidepressants. Her pain started about five years ago.

When I touched her muscles, it was obvious to me that she was dehydrated. Hers did not feel like well-hydrated tissue. Her posture was quite poor, which indicated numerous muscle imbalances. It took me about 30 minutes to rebalance her muscles and bring her body back into alignment. Her pain levels decreased immediately. I explained to her that her pain would not completely go away until her tissues were rehydrated. Improved fluid intake would most likely also help with depression and brain fog. I told her it could take up to 8 weeks to rehydrate.

I showed her the Wellness Plan and instructed her to be consistent doing the plan every day. I gave her advice on how to rehydrate her body.

I saw her two months later and she reported she was greatly improved, although she still had some pain. Sometimes the rehydration and the Wellness Plan take a little longer to work.

Another month after that, she reported that she was 90% pain-free. There were many days when there was no pain at all. She has since stopped taking pain-killers and antidepressants and her mood has greatly improved.

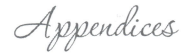

CAUTION

With the following exercises, never stretch into a painful position. You will achieve better results by being gentle.

The goal is not to stretch as far as possible but to slightly increase range of motion.

Done consistently, the results can be dramatic and permanent.

Nothing should ever hurt while doing these exercises.

If pain occurs during an exercise, try the stretch or position more gently. If it still hurts, skip that exercise for now and continue with the ones that don't hurt.

If you are not getting better in a few weeks of doing these exercises, please check with your health care provider for more insight into your condition.

Appendix A:
Proper Sitting, Computer and Driving Positions

Proper Sitting Position

Sit with a pillow or a small rolled-up towel placed in the lumbar curve. This is just above the belt line. It is important that the pillow is the right thickness. Every chair and every body needs a different thickness. The pillow should be thick enough to bring your head back over your shoulders and open the chest. If the pillow is too thick it will hurt and if it is not thick enough your head will be forward of your body. The correct position allows the skeleton to support your body and should feel comfortable. This will contribute to overall good posture and reduced back and neck pain. If this is painful, disregard for now.

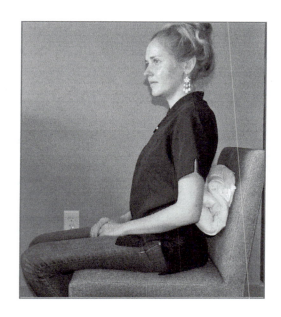

Improper Sitting Position

This typical unsupported position can cause muscle tension in the low back, upper back, neck and shoulders. This position can also make the hips uneven and lead to disc problems. In this position, your muscles are working to hold you up, creating tension and pain.

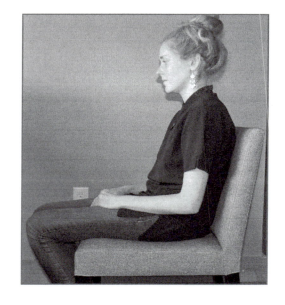

Proper Computer Position

When sitting at your desk, keep your elbows by your side. Arms should be bent about 90 degrees. To find this position, stand normally with your arms at your side. Bend the elbows to 90 degrees. That should be how it looks and feels when you are sitting. The computer monitor should be eye height and straight in front of you so you are not bending your neck. Feet should be flat on the floor or on a foot rest. Dangling feet can cause low back pain and poor circulation.

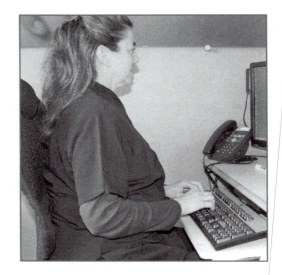

Improper Computer Position

This position can cause muscle tension in the jaw, shoulder and neck. Do not reach for the mouse or keyboard.

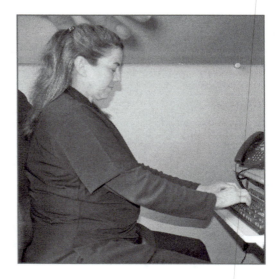

Proper Driving Position

When driving, use your pillow or towel and keep your elbows at your side. Hands should be at about the 8:00 and 4:00 positions. This position allows your bones to support your body, avoids excessive muscle tension in neck and shoulders and helps to avoid potential trauma to the face if your air bags deploy. Many states now teach their new drivers to hold the wheel at 8:00 and 4:00 as a safety precaution to prevent injury from airbag deployment.

WARNING: If you do not feel safe driving at the 4:00 and 8:00 hand positions, then drive the way you normally do. It is better to have sore muscles and be safe. If you do feel comfortable driving at 4:00 and 8:00, you will find that this is a much better ergonomic position.

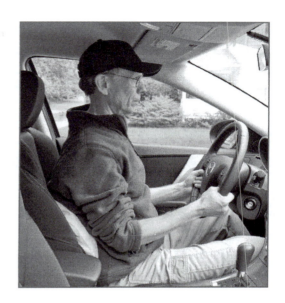

Improper Driving Position

Driving with hands at the 10:00 and 2:00 positions can cause muscle tension in the upper back, shoulders and neck.

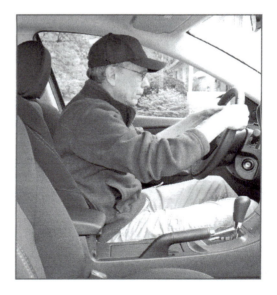

Appendix B:
Three Stretches to Balance the Pelvis

These stretches will usually bring your pelvis into alignment. They will ensure there is no abnormal strain on your hip joints, knees or feet and they correct the most common imbalances in the pelvis. Perform these three stretches 1 to 3 times per day to keep your hips in alignment. These stretches should be done gently and should not cause any pain. Breathe normally throughout these exercises – don't hold your breath!

Quadratus Lumborum Stretch

Stand up straight with your legs slightly apart. Raise your arm on one side so that your fingers are pointing towards the ceiling and slowly bend towards the opposite side, reaching with your raised hand and arm until you feel a stretch along the side of your upper body. Rest the non-reaching hand on your leg. Hold 30 seconds while breathing normally. Repeat on the other side.

Feel the stretch here ➝

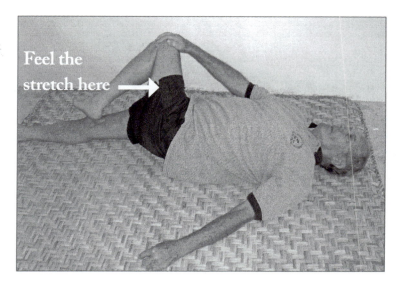

Feel the stretch here →

Abductor Stretch

Lie on your back. Bend one leg and place the sole of the foot on the opposite leg. Gently use your hand to pull your bent knee towards the floor. Feel the stretch on the outside of the upper leg and in the buttocks. Without letting the bent knee move, gently push the knee towards the ceiling, resisting with your hand, for 5 seconds. Now pull the leg into a deeper stretch towards the floor. Hold for 30 seconds. Repeat on the other side.

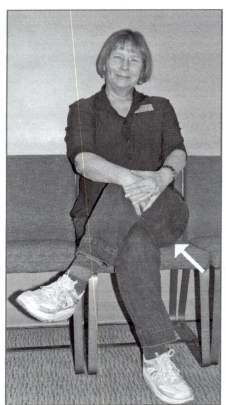

Feel the stretch here

Modified Version: Sit in a chair and cross one leg over the other. This will gently stretch your abductor muscles on the outside of the upper leg. Do not perform this exercise if your legs 'fall asleep.'

Quadriceps Stretch

Hold onto the back of a chair or put your hand on a wall to help keep your balance. Reach back with one hand to grasp the foot and bring the heel towards the buttocks. Feel the stretch in the front of the upper leg. Push your foot gently into your hand for 5 seconds. Bring the heel closer to the buttocks to deepen the stretch and hold for 30 seconds. Repeat on other side.

Modified version: Place the top of the foot and the lower leg on a chair or sofa to achieve this stretch. Repeat on other side.

Feel the stretch here →

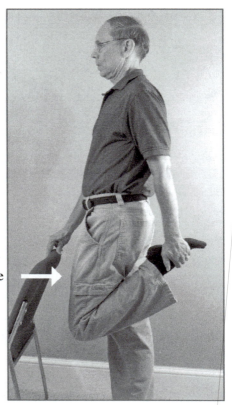

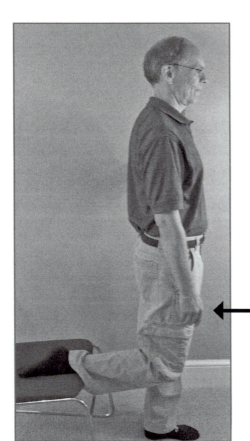

← Feel the stretch here

Appendix C:
Three Neck Stretches

These three stretches release the muscles in the neck and bring relief to the area. They also allow increased blood flow and oxygen to the brain. Try doing these three stretches in a warm shower every morning as the stretches work even better when the neck tissue is warm. Do these exercises 1 to 3 times a day. Always work gently and slowly.

Back of the Neck Stretch

With hands at the back of the head, pull head forward until a slight stretch is felt. Gently push backward into your hands for 5 seconds but do not let the head move. Now pull forward into a deeper stretch. Repeat a few times as long as it feels good. This will stretch the muscles along the back of your neck.

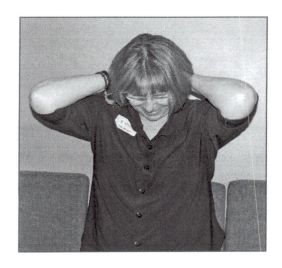

Side of the Neck Stretch

With your hand, pull your head to one side until a slight stretch is felt. Reach with the opposite hand towards the floor throughout the exercise. Gently push your head into your hand for 5 seconds but do not let the head move. Now pull head to the side into a deeper stretch. Repeat a few times as long as it feels good. Repeat on the other side. This exercise stretches the muscles on the side of your neck.

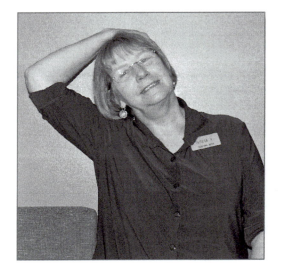

Front of the Neck Stretch

Turn your head to one side to look over your shoulder until you feel a slight stretch in your neck. Place your hand on your cheek and gently try to turn back to center, resisting with your hand against your cheek for 5 seconds. Do not let the head move. Then turn your head into a deeper stretch towards the first direction. Repeat a few times as long as it feels good. Repeat on other side. This exercise stretches the muscles on the front of your neck.

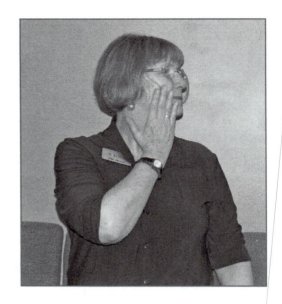

Appendix D:
Jaw

Slacken the Jaw

Gently push the lower jaw to one side and hold for two minutes. Repeat on other side.

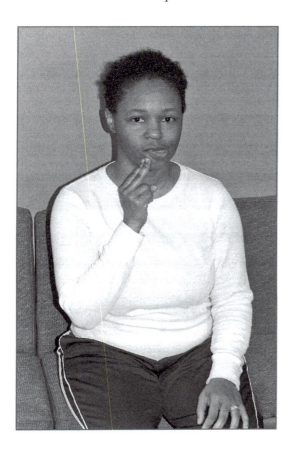 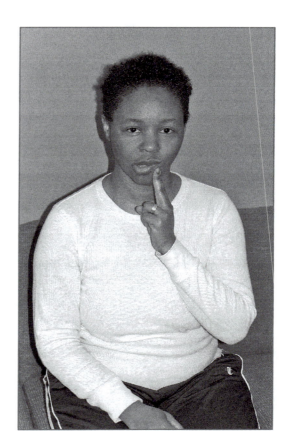

Appendix E:
Shoulders

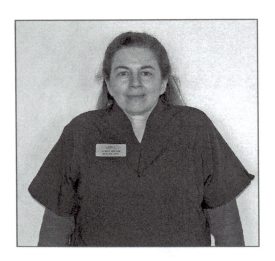

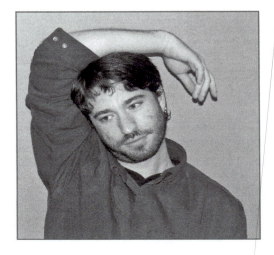

Shoulder Shrugs

Gently squeeze your shoulders up towards your ears and hold for about 10 seconds. Repeat many times throughout the day.

Slacken the Shoulders

Place arm on top of head and let it rest in that position with the head tilted towards the painful side. Hold for at least two minutes. This position will relieve tension in the shoulders especially the upper trapezius and levator scapula. Do this any time you feel any tension in your shoulders or neck. Do not do this if it hurts to put your arm on top of your head.

Strengthen Rhomboids

From a standing position with your arms at your side, raise your arms in front of you so they are parallel to the ground. Make a fist with both hands and pull back so that your elbows are at your side. Squeeze the shoulder blades together for 5 seconds using a motion like you are rowing a boat. This will help to shorten and strengthen the muscles between the shoulder blades thus training the muscles to bring the head over the shoulders, improving the posture and reducing the strain on the neck. Do this 10 times, 3 times a day.

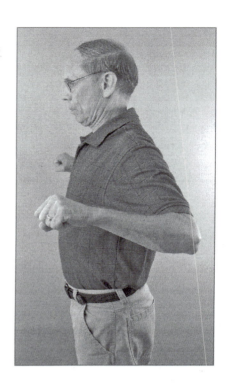

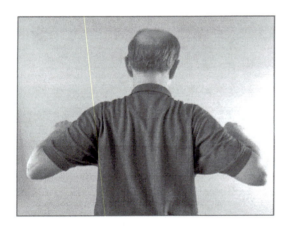

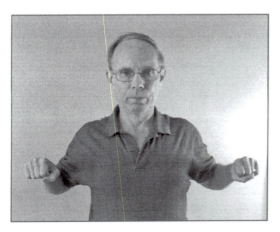

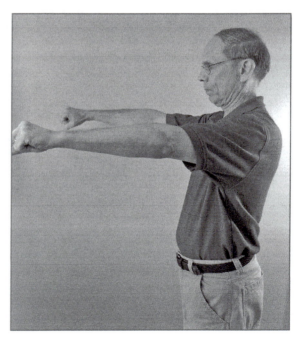

Appendix F:
Chest Exercises

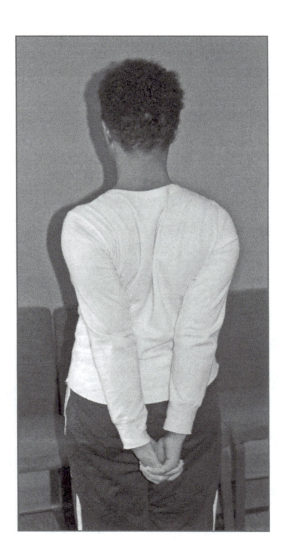

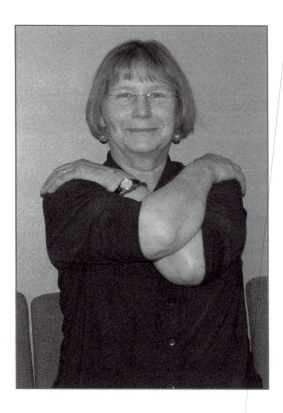

Slacken the Chest

Place each hand on the opposite shoulder as if hugging yourself. Totally relax and hold the position for two minutes.

Stretch the Chest

Squeeze shoulder blades together gently. Hold for at least two minutes. This will stretch the chest muscles and release tension between the shoulder blades and the muscle known as the rhomboids.

Appendix G:
Arm and Hand Exercises

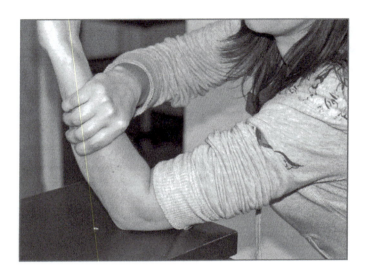

Elbow Tendon Release

Gently push the tissue of the forearm towards the elbow. Hold at least two minutes.

Slacken the Thumb

Gently squeeze your thumb and palm together so that your little finger and thumb are touching. Hold at least two minutes.

If you are treating Carpal Tunnel Syndrome, keep your wrist straight. A bent wrist could bring on numbness and tingling.

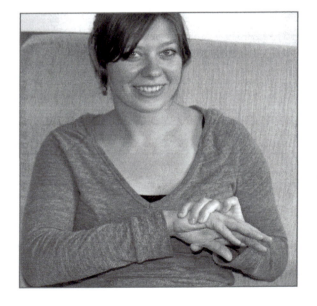

Slacken and Stretch the Forearm – two directions

Gently twist your palm so your thumb faces down. This will release tension in your elbow and wrist. Hold at least two minutes. Then twist the arm the other way and hold for two minutes. If any of these twists bring on the symptoms do not do these exercises until your symptoms dissipate.

If you are treating Carpal Tunnel Syndrome, keep your wrist straight. A bent wrist could bring on numbness and tingling.

For Tennis Elbow, the wrist should be slightly bent backward.

For Golfer's elbow, the wrist should be slightly bent forward.

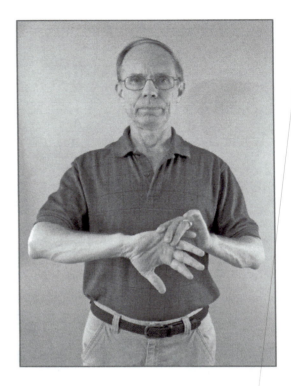

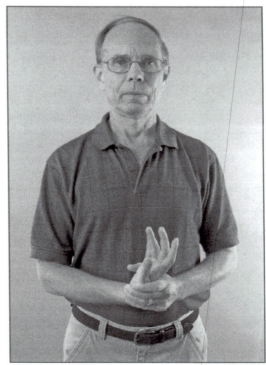

Appendix H:
Hip and Buttocks Exercises

Slacken the Hip Flexors (Psoas and Quadriceps)

Lie on your back on the floor. Bend at the hip 90 degrees and at the knees 90 degrees. Rest the lower legs on a chair or sofa. Relax in this position for at least two minutes.

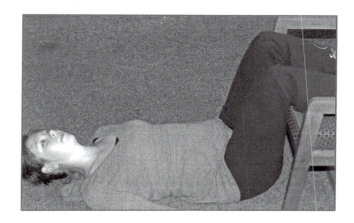

Slacken the Piriformis (Half-Frog)

Lie on your stomach. Bend one knee and bring that leg about half-way up along the floor so that the thigh is at a right angle (or slightly less) to your torso (half-frog). Hold at least two minutes. This will release tension in your low back and the piriformis. Repeat on other side.

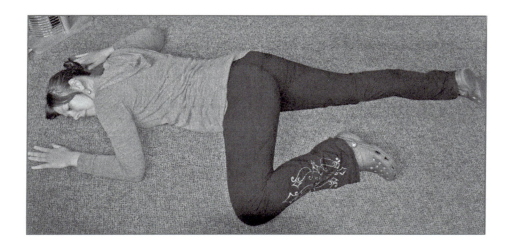

Appendix I:
Inner Thigh Exercises

Slacken the Inside Thighs (Adductors)

Sit with thighs spiraled in (pigeon-toed.) Relax in this position for at least two minutes. Sitting with your legs and feet slightly turned in will take the strain off the lower back, knees and groin. Do not walk or stand like this – do the exercise only when sitting.

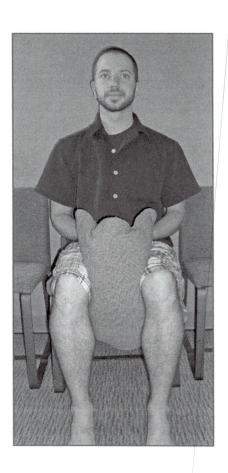

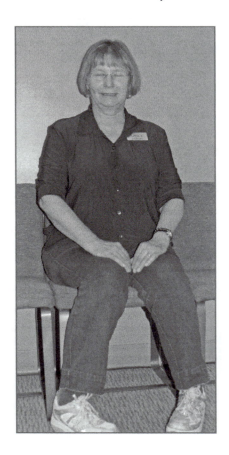

Strengthen the Inside Thighs (Adductors)

Sit in a chair. Fold a bed pillow in half and place it between the knees. You can also use a small ball. Squeeze the knees together for about 5 seconds. Do ten of these squeezes and then rest for a minute. Do another ten squeezes and rest again for one minute. Continue in this manner until you can do about 5 sets of 10. This will strengthen the muscles on the inside of your legs and begin to reduce your symptoms.

Appendix J:
Lower Leg Exercises

Slacken the Calf

Sit in a chair and place the sore foot or calf on the opposite thigh. Gently bend your foot giving yourself a big arch. Hold that position for two minutes. This puts the calf muscle, the bottom of the foot and the Achilles tendon into a slackened position and gives almost immediate relief. In this case, more often is better.

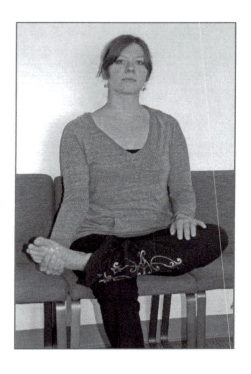

Stretch the Calf

Stand on the edge of a step and let the heels gently drop toward the floor. Hold for ten seconds. Do not stretch too deeply. If this hurts, the stretch is too deep.

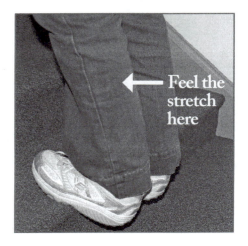

Feel the stretch here

Achilles Tendon Release

Place foot on the opposite thigh and gently push the two ends of the tendon together. Hold for two minutes. Do this five times a day.

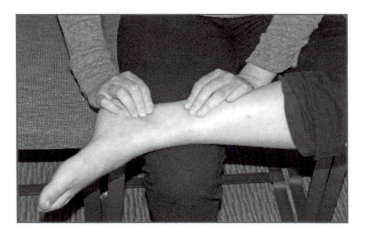

For more information, please visit Lee's website at
www.LeeAlbert.com

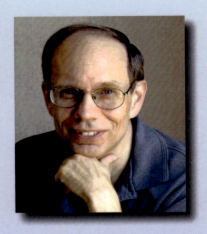

LEE ALBERT, NMT, creator of Integrated Positional Therapy (IPT), is a nationally recognized expert in neuro-muscular pain relief. For over 25 years he has helped people learn how to live pain-free using the tools and techniques of IPT. He treats patients one-on-one at the Kripalu Center for Yoga & Health in Lenox, MA and conducts training seminars in IPT. Lee also consults with businesses on ergonomic training for employees to reduce workplace injuries.

www.LeeAlbert.com

DUDLEY COURT PRESS
SONOITA, ARIZONA, U.S.A.
www.DudleyCourtPress.com

DO YOU SUFFER from chronic or occasional headaches, neck and shoulder pain, low back pain or knee pain?

Have you been diagnosed with fibromyalgia, tennis or golfer's elbow, carpal tunnel syndrome, TMJ, plantar fasciitis, thoracic outlet syndrome or sciatica?

Would you like to cure your neuromuscular pain without surgery or drugs?

Live Pain-free offers a practical, proven, easy-to-follow program (Integrated Positional Therapy) to reduce and even eliminate chronic muscular pain in only minutes a day through simple exercises and movements that anyone can do.

Developed by neuromuscular therapist Lee Albert, NMT, Integrated Positional Therapy (IPT) incorporates techniques such as Strain/Counterstrain, Muscle Energy Technique, stretching and home care to re-align the body's structure and relieve pain caused by structural imbalances. IPT effectively treats pain patterns caused by injury, stress, repetitive strain, postural distortion and chronic neuromuscular conditions.

Written in a clear and user-friendly manner, *Live Pain-free* includes detailed descriptions and photos to make the exercises very easy to follow at home. The book offers valuable information on basic body care along with individual treatment protocols for eleven of the most common conditions that cause people to seek medical attention:

- Headaches
- Neck and shoulder pain
- Low back pain
- Knee pain
- Fibromyalgia
- Tennis and golfer's elbow
- Carpal tunnel syndrome
- TMJ
- Plantar fasciitis
- Thoracic outlet syndrome
- Sciatica

Thousands of patients and students from all over the world have benefitted from Integrated Positional Therapy. Now you can benefit in your own home from the same simple program for permanent relief from neuromuscular pain *without surgery or drugs*.

$29.95
ISBN 978-0-9831383-1-0